# Bodies and Lives in Victorian England

This volume offers an overview of what it was like to be female and to live and die in Victorian England (c. 1837–1901), by situating this experience within the scientific and social contexts of the times.

With a temporal focus on women's life experience, the book moves from childhood and youth, through puberty and adolescence, to pregnancy, birth, and motherhood, into senescence. Drawing on osteological sources, medical discourses, and examples from the literature and cultural history of the period, alongside social and environmental data derived from ethnographic and archival investigations, the authors explore the experience of being female in the Victorian era for women across classes. In synthesizing current research on demographic statistics, maternal morbidity and mortality, and bioarchaeological evidence on patterns of aging and death, they analyze how changing social ideals, cultural and environmental variability, shifting economies, and evolving medical and scientific understanding about the body combined to shape female health and identity in the nineteenth century. Victorian women faced a variety of challenges, including changing attitudes regarding appropriate behavior, social roles, and beauty standards, while grappling with new understandings of the role played by gender and sexuality in shaping women's lives from youth to old age.

The book concludes by considering the relevance of how Victorian narratives of womanhood and the experience of being female have influenced perceptions of female health and cultural constructions of identity today.

**Pamela K. Stone** is Visiting Associate Professor of Anthropology at Hampshire College, Amherst, MA, USA.

**Lise Shapiro Sanders** is Professor of English Literature and Cultural Studies at Hampshire College, Amherst, MA, USA.

**Bodies and Lives**
**Series Editor:** Anna Osterholtz

**Bodies and Lives in Victorian England**
Science, Sexuality, and the Affliction of Being Female
*Pamela K. Stone and Lise Shapiro Sanders*

https://www.routledge.com/Bodies-and-Lives/book-series/BODLIV

# Bodies and Lives in Victorian England

## Science, Sexuality, and the Affliction of Being Female

**Pamela K. Stone and Lise Shapiro Sanders**

Routledge
Taylor & Francis Group
LONDON AND NEW YORK

First published 2021
by Routledge
2 Park Square, Milton Park, Abingdon, Oxon OX14 4RN

and by Routledge
52 Vanderbilt Avenue, New York, NY 10017

Routledge is an imprint of the Taylor & Francis Group, an informa business



*British Library Cataloguing-in-Publication Data*
A catalogue record for this book is available from the British Library

*Library of Congress Cataloging-in-Publication Data*
Names: Stone, Pamela K, author. | Sanders, Lise Shapiro, 1970- author.
Title: Bodies and lives in Victorian England: science, sexuality, and the affliction of being female / Pamela K. Stone and Lise Shapiro Sanders.
Description: Abingdon, Oxon; New York, NY: Routledge, 2021. |
Series: Bodies and lives | Includes bibliographical references and index.
Identifiers: LCCN 2020017824 (print) | LCCN 2020017825 (ebook) |
ISBN 9780367026110 (hardback) | ISBN 9780429398735 (ebook)
Subjects: LCSH: Women–Great Britain–History–19th century. | Sex–Great Britain–History–19th century. | Sex role–Great Britain–History–19th century. | Great Britain–Social life and customs–History–19th century.
Classification: LCC HQ1593 .S846 2021 (print) | LCC HQ1593 (ebook) |
DDC 305.40941/09034–dc23
LC record available at https://lccn.loc.gov/2020017824
LC ebook record available at https://lccn.loc.gov/2020017825

ISBN: 978-0-367-02611-0 (hbk)
ISBN: 978-0-429-39873-5 (ebk)

Typeset in Times New Roman
by Deanta Global Publishing Services, Chennai, India

**To our Hampshire College mentors, colleagues, and students**

# Contents

# Figures

# Acknowledgments

This book was inspired by our co-taught course "Sex, Science, and the Victorian Body," which we have been teaching at Hampshire College since 2011. The course, in turn, emerged as a result of conversations with our student, Frances Campbell, who crafted an interdisciplinary undergraduate concentration in women's studies with a focus on bodies in Victorian culture. For these reasons, and as a result of our shared experience of being both alumnae and faculty members at the same institution, this is an eminently Hampshire-esque project. We are indebted to our faculty mentors and colleagues, as well as several generations of students, whose insights, questions, and projects have immeasurably enriched this work. We are also grateful to the staff of a number of archives and special collections, including the British Library, the Elizabeth Garrett Anderson Gallery, the Florence Nightingale Museum, the Royal College of Obstetricians and Gynaecologists, the Wellcome Collection, and the Women's Library at the London School of Economics. In the references at the end of each chapter, we hope to have signaled our debt to the rich scholarship in biocultural anthropology, cultural and social history, literary studies, and other disciplines that make up the thriving interdisciplinary field of Bioarchaeology and Victorian Studies. We especially appreciate the comments of three anonymous reviewers, whose suggestions were very useful. Any errors are, of course, our own.

Pamela K. Stone would like to thank Dr. Anna Osterholtz for inviting her to be a part of this series on bodies and lives, and Dr. Lise Shapiro Sanders for joining her on the collaborative creation of this text. She would also like to acknowledge her mentors, colleagues, and students, from Hampshire College and beyond, who have consistently challenged, supported, and collaborated with her to develop and consider the larger theoretical, social, and cultural contexts in which bodies are assessed—among them Debra Martin, Kay Johnson, Loretta Ross, Jennifer Hamilton, Ventura Perez, Hanna D. Polasky, and Claira Ralston for her wonderful drawings—and as always, her friends and family, especially Jim, Riley, and Tanner.

Lise Shapiro Sanders would like to thank Dr. Pamela K. Stone for the initial inspiration behind this book, and for facilitating such a productive collaboration. She is grateful to her Five College Victorianist colleagues, and the members of Cathy Luna's online writing group, for their unfailing encouragement. She would also like to thank her students—among them Zara Cannon-Mohammed, Gabriel Horvath, Monique Jacques, Emily Murphy, Lanah Swindle, and Blair Talbot—as well as faculty and staff colleagues at Hampshire and elsewhere. Lastly, she is thankful for the support of friends and family, especially her parents, who read the manuscript in draft form, and Eric and Henry, who never seem to mind yet another conversation about the fascinations of the Victorian era.

# 1 Introduction

## Why a Book on Victorian Women's Bodies?

*Bodies and Lives in Victorian England: Science, Sexuality, and the Affliction of Being Female* offers a broad overview of what it was like to be female and to live and die in Victorian England (c. 1837–1901). With a temporal focus on women's life experience, this interdisciplinary study moves from childhood and youth, through puberty and adolescence, to pregnancy, birth, and motherhood, into senescence. Reviewing the literature on skeletal remains, and drawing on medical discourses and examples from the literature and cultural history of the period alongside social and environmental data derived from ethnographic and archival investigations, we explore the experience of being female in the Victorian era for women across classes. In synthesizing current research on demographic statistics, maternal morbidity and mortality, and bioarchaeological evidence on patterns of aging and death, we analyze how changing social ideals, cultural and environmental variability, shifting economies, and evolving medical and scientific understanding about the body combined to shape female health (wellness and illness) and identity in the nineteenth century. Victorian women faced a variety of challenges, including changing attitudes regarding appropriate behavior, social roles, and beauty standards, while grappling with new understandings of the role played by gender and sexuality in shaping women's lives from youth to old age. The book concludes by considering the relevance of how Victorian narratives of womanhood and the experience of being female have influenced perceptions of female health and cultural constructions of identity today.

Two unique features set this text apart from other current scholarship in Victorian history, anthropology, and literary and cultural studies. First, the focus on *women's* bodies and lives enables a narrowed scope that attends specifically to questions of female physiology, health, and wellness, without taking the male body as the norm. Second, the interdisciplinary focus on reading science and culture together—through a biocultural approach, defined in detail below—facilitates a set of intersecting questions and perspectives that would otherwise be elided. In the past 30 years, for example, numerous books have been published in the field of Victorian cultural studies, many with a focus on fashion and the body, tropes of femininity, and women's compliance with, or deviance from, constructed social norms and ideologies of gender in this period. However, none of these texts has adopted the biocultural approach that is a hallmark of this book, and none has examined the Victorian female body using osteological and medical data alongside cultural and historical analysis. The existing scholarship examining the body against the backdrop of industrial/political economies and their implications for Victorian women tends to focus on narrowly defined aspects of life in the Victorian era, such as asylums and mental illness, and fashion (corsets), femininity, and beauty; but often with little or no attention to the impact on the skeletal body, anatomy and physiology, and women's health. Outside of academia, many websites and blogs explore women's bodily experience in the Victorian era, but few offer clear information on the sources of their knowledge. In the most egregious examples, women are sensationalized for their roles in the horrific state of the asylum and their place in the world of fashion and beauty; in these cases, women take the stage as the deviant, exotic, and erotic. But women's everyday lives and lived experiences, and the health issues they suffered as a result of cultural transformations that directly impacted their bodies, are often not discussed. This trend holds true as well for the majority of scholarly articles and research papers in anthropology, as they may address some of the skeletal consequences of changing medical and scientific practices, but they focus largely on disease pathologies. They therefore miss the opportunity to draw on larger cultural and ideological frameworks to explore the role, position, and impact of rapidly transforming social and economic landscapes, alongside changing approaches to medicine and health, on the construction of femininity and the experience of being female during the Victorian era.

In this introductory chapter, we first define the key terms we use throughout the text, among them sex, gender, and sexuality; biocultural approaches and bioarchaeological methods; and the value of using microhistories to elucidate the historical and social contexts for women's lived experience in the nineteenth century. We then address the theoretical frameworks for our book, among them Foucauldian discourse theory, theories of structural violence and embodiment, gender and queer studies, and critical race studies. Lastly, we offer a brief historical overview of the Victorian era, with particular attention to the significance of the industrial revolution; class difference and struggle; racial difference, the imperial project, and the effects of colonialism on England and its "others"; and new conceptions of sex, gender, and sexuality—all with an eye toward women's health, wellness and illness, and the cultural role of the female body. Our introduction concludes with an outline of the book's four main chapters, which trace a temporal overview of women's life experience, and a brief discussion of our conclusions and opportunities for further research.

### *Defining Terms: Sex, Gender, and Sexuality*

First and foremost, it is important to delimit the scope of our project, particularly with respect to sex, gender, and sexuality. When we use the term "sex," we mean the biological elements that differentiate male and female physiology, namely the primary and secondary sexual characteristics, that lead to an individual being assigned the sex of "male" or "female" at birth. "Gender," by contrast, is a much more complex set of individual and cultural definitions and associations, to do with aspects of identity, behavior, and an individual's relationship to society. And "sexuality" entails all the aspects of human sexual behavior, from sexual orientation to the way one experiences sexual pleasure. "Sex," therefore, has to do with biological (anatomical and chromosomal) differences, whereas "gender" has to do with the way one identifies, and in many cases the way one is identified by culture and society.

But sex, gender, and sexuality do not necessarily fit such binary definitions. The binary distinction between "male" and female" in the determination of what sex an individual is assigned at birth does not take into account the wide range of anatomical and chromosomal variations in human sexual identity; hence the use of the term "intersex" to represent sexual categories that do not fall neatly into "male" or "female" (Fausto-Sterling 1993, 2000). And "gender" is far more complex than simply identifying as a girl or a boy, a man or a woman. People whose gender identity more or less accords with the sex they were assigned at birth are termed "cisgender"; people whose gender identity does not align with the sex they were assigned at birth use the term "transgender" or simply "trans" to represent their gender identity. Gender-non-conforming, genderfluid, genderqueer, and nonbinary are all terms used to describe the wide array of gender identities and expressions experienced by people today. Sexual orientation, likewise, can be considered on a spectrum rather than as a binary of homosexual or heterosexual.[1] And since the publication of Judith Butler's influential text *Gender Trouble* in 1990, even the conventional distinctions between sex and gender have been shown to be "troubled" by the fact that sex does not exist before or without gender. Butler's argument regarding the performativity of gender has played an important role in the development of fields such as queer and transgender studies, and has opened up key questions about the nature of sex, gender, and sexuality in contemporary culture as well as in history.

In the Victorian period, sex and gender—and sexuality—were subject to cultural and societal expectations that perpetuated a set of what we would now call gender-normative definitions of male and female, which aligned an individual's assigned sex with their gender identity and made it difficult for people to adopt alternative modes of gender expression. In an intensely homophobic era in which male homosexuality was not only culturally proscribed but liable to criminal prosecution, and in which (because of cultural assumptions about women's sexuality or the lack thereof) female homosexuality was practically inconceivable, it was also difficult—if not impossible—for gay, lesbian, and queer people to openly express their sexual orientation without fear of reprisal. Nonetheless, as scholarship in the history of sexuality has shown, Victorians embraced a wide range of gendered and sexual identities, acts, and practices that contradict the popular perception of Victorian culture as prudish, repressed, and sexually inactive (Marcus 1966; Foucault 1976; Sedgwick 1985, 1990). In fact, the Victorian period is one of the most fascinating eras for the study of changing conceptions of gender and sexuality, as we explore at greater length below.

For the purposes of this book, when we use the phrase "Victorian women," we mean people who defined themselves as women in the nineteenth century, some of whom may or may not have identified with the sex they were assigned at birth. When we use the phrase "the female body," we intend to signify those elements of sex that are associated with the skeletal, anatomical, and biological definitions of "female." For the most part, although exceptions do exist in the scholarly and archival record, this means that the association of the terms "women" and "female bodies" presumes a cisgendered understanding of the relationship between sex and gender in the Victorian period—a restricted view, to be sure. However, contemporary scholars are working within a set of complex and intersecting discourses and changing definitions of sexuality in nineteenth-century England, and we still have much to learn about the ways in which Victorians navigated their own understandings of sex, gender, and sexuality.

### *Microhistories and Historical Contexts*

A microhistory approach is one in which smaller units of research (events, communities, settlements, even an individual) are explored in order to understand larger, macro-level questions in historical context (Joyner 1999; Lepore 2001). By concentrating on Victorian England and women's lived experience across classes, and examining critical life stages from birth to death, we can explore how the rapidly developing fields of human science and social analysis become deeply entwined with political ideologies and meaning. Victorian scientists, largely male, white, and from the elite classes, elaborated what they saw as clear-cut distinctions of sex, gender, race, and social status, which in turn resulted in the construction of "normal" and "deviant" bodies that shaped legal and social understandings. In particular, Victorian science and medicine created a narrative of racial hierarchy and difference that took culturally constructed distinctions as biologically determined. These frameworks need to be understood as contingent rather than universal.

### *Biocultural Approaches and Bioarchaeology*

In addition to engaging in microhistorical analysis, we also employ a biocultural approach in developing our analysis of women's bodies and lives in the Victorian period. This approach requires us to consider multiple lines of inquiry that engage both social and biological understandings of what it means to be female in this era. In this text, we consider how evolving scientific inquiry into human variation is layered onto the lived experiences of people during the nineteenth century, while also considering how people embodied the narratives that science was developing in relation to social expectations. For example, the impact of corsets on the health and wellness of young women did not involve a single factor, but rather constituted a set of biological and social implications for young women that placed them at higher risk for sickness and potential death (as we address in greater detail in Chapter 3). While much of the cultural and biological evidence for our analysis can be gleaned from texts, diaries, medical reports, and many other sources for this time frame, we also consider scholarship that uses a bioarchaeological approach, looking directly at the skeletal body, to understand women's health, wellness, and illness in the nineteenth century.

Bioarchaeological analysis offers a direct transcript of life. When examined in broader contexts, skeletal traces of health and disease can shed light on the complexity of the lived experience that may not have been articulated within the written literature (Geller 2016). For a study of female lives and bodies in the past, it is not only crucial that multiple lines of inquiry (skeletal, ethnohistoric, archaeological) are used to guide the discussion of gender, ideology, and power; it is also vital to ask whose bodies are being examined, and to what end this informs our understanding of lived experience, for all classes of women. We recognize that modern, Western conceptions of human experience have been influenced by nineteenth-century constructions of normative identity and gender roles, and we use an intersectional theoretical approach to engage critically with Victorian ideological frameworks. In so doing, we benefit from an interdisciplinary mode of inquiry that brings together scientific and cultural methods of analysis, expanding the types of questions that may be asked about the past and creating a holistic view of what it meant to be female in Victorian England.

## Theoretical Frameworks

This book uses several key theoretical frameworks. Using structural violence theory and theories of embodiment, we examine the relationship between individuals and the society in which they lived, paying particular attention to the way traces of the past can be found on the body. In our analysis of race, gender, sex and sexuality, and class, we take an intersectional approach, striving to put a variety of elements into play in our understanding of the bodies and lived experiences covered by the scope of our study. The following section defines each of these theories and provides examples from the period under discussion to elucidate their usefulness for this analysis.

### *Structural Violence Theory*

The phrase "structural violence" expresses the concept that social structures (economic, political, medical, and legal systems) exert power and pressure over individuals and communities to perform in expected ways, producing inequalities that result in preventable suffering (Galtung 1969; Martin and Harrod 2012; Lewis 2019). While it is often assumed that structural violence is inflicted on disenfranchised groups, structural violence can impact people from all classes and ethnicities, as it requires adherence to the dominant system, which in turn has a disproportionately negative impact on the particular individual, group, or community that does not conform, or is deemed deviant. Galtung (1969), who first coined the concept of structural violence, framed it as the root cause of the differences between people's potential reality and their actual circumstances. If we consider the male-dominated medical system and the medicalization of childbirth, and its role in shaping increased rates of female morbidity and mortality, we can see the role of structural violence in the policing of the birth process. Prior to the nineteenth century, birth was a female-centered, home experience, attended by midwives, whose training was predicated on their own experiences and a long history of attending births. While today most people safely give birth under the care of highly trained physicians in hospitals, it is the shift in the Victorian era from hearth and home to lying-in hospitals—staffed by doctors with little understanding of infectious transmission and dominated by treatments that focused on painkillers and the tools of birth (clinical spaces, forceps, scalpels)—that resulted in a dramatic upswing of childbed fevers and maternal deaths (Loudon 1997; Stone 2009, 2016). This new hospital-based system most dramatically affected the elite classes, as medicine was seen as cosmopolitan and access to care was a status symbol, while also functioning as a means to distance women from their own bodies (Jordan 1993; Davis-Floyd and Sargent 1997; Stone 2009). The Victorian medicalization of childbirth also set the tone for new models of control over the female reproductive body, exemplifying how structural violence becomes built into the medical system, and how its impact on female health and autonomy becomes normalized and left unquestioned. Current scholarship in anthropology considers the ways in which death as a result of childbirth has been systematically misunderstood, producing a narrative that female bodies are fragile and in need of medical care, neglecting birthing traditions and the far longer history of successful birth experiences. The lack of attention to women's own experiences and processes of childbirth has resulted in an ingrained system of structural violence that dismisses female bodily autonomy and women's biological ability to give birth.

Using structural violence theory as a framework in the examination and interpretation of past lived experiences in bioarchaeology requires us to employ a biocultural system of inquiry to consider how individuals, through their bodies, are implicated in social expectations and the performance of cultural norms. Adherence to a single birth model offers a case in point: with a structural violence approach, we can understand better why women give over their understanding of how their bodies work, participating in the dominant view of childbirth as a traumatic experience best undertaken in a hospital environment. Yet most often, we think of violence in terms of experiences that are direct, visible, and cause recognizable damage, such as an immediate violent action (a punch to the face) or a long-term, chronic expression of domination (as in the suffering of individuals in a city under siege). As in the case of the birthing system, some violence is more difficult to trace, or has been made part of the normal fabric of the cultural environment, which means that it can be virtually invisible if we don't know how to understand its markers. For example, research has shown that living with a lifetime of racism puts African-American women at higher risk for complications such as preterm births, low birth-weight, and stillbirths (Murrell 1996; Lu and Halfon 2003; Collins et al. 2004; Mustillo et al. 2004). Having been subjected to racism over the course of their lifetimes, African-American women have suffered the effects of long-term and chronic discrimination, and this causes physiological disruptions that result in these high-risk birth situations (Collins et al. 2004; Giurgescu et al. 2011). Thus, to assume that the absence of direct evidence means there is an absence of violence may result in missing the larger social dynamics influencing the experience of the individual, the social group, or even the state, within the particular culture being examined. Interpretations of indirect violence are complicated within the analysis of the bioarchaeological record as they can be hard to identify, particularly when there is an absence of cultural artifacts, written records, and ethnographic analogies. Thus, the analysis of structural violence can be hindered, as it is often invisible or attributed to other types of disparity, which are often ascribed to women and children.

In the case of Victorian women, we have a vast array of documentation, ranging from primary textual evidence to osteological data, which can be used to understand the role of the white elite class as the central driving force in the structural violence of the period. First, as we discuss at length in Chapter 2, Victorian science centered the elite white male body as normal within all aspects of the social, economic, medical, and legal systems. The systemic normalization of the male body both produced and was produced by a Victorian patriarchal system centered on male dominance and control, with women being seen as weak, fragile, and less able, and having to perform in certain ways in order to be acceptable within the social order. Victorian cultural codes of behavior and civility, which were developed to reinforce the white European male as more evolved than all others, served to further support these scientific and social constructions. These deeply entrenched Victorian ideas were central to how all aspects of human variation were being understood: race, sex and gender, socioeconomic status, and even assumptions of beauty were used to reinforce hegemonic power dynamics. For women these ideological discourses resulted in cultural expectations for dress and behavior that often resulted in long-term chronic stressors across class. As scholars have noted, it is often the elite who script the systems of structural violence, but this does not mean they are impervious to the stressors and consequences of their expectations (Galtung 1969, 1990; Farmer et al. 2004; Stone 2012).

At the roots of structural violence are assumptions of established order that monitor, to different degrees, the behaviors, attitudes, and conditions that are set by those in power. Conforming to social expectations keeps the system operational and somewhat invisible in the way in which it controls the population; in this way, structural violence accords well with the concept of hegemony, a term developed by Italian theorist Antonio Gramsci to describe how individuals and societies participate in dominant social systems and consent to their own oppression within such systems. In contrast, deviance from the system may result in direct and highly visible consequences. In the Victorian era, elite white women participated intentionally and unintentionally in the power structures that underpinned the structural violence of the era (Campbell 2012). Their adherence to social expectations was central in enforcing codes for feminine behavior, even when they resulted in compromising women's health, keeping them from being educated, and in many ways regulating women to be the property of their husbands. The Victorian feminist movement, discussed in Chapters 2 and 3, took on precisely these questions in challenging existing medical, educational, and legal modes of discrimination based on an ideological narrative that privileged, and pigeonholed, women as "the weaker sex." The embedded structural violence of Victorian patriarchy rendered women unable to participate in society at the same level as men, producing and reinforcing the narrative of female disability that frames how we think about female agency in the past and the present. Uncovering the layers of structural violence to understand the lived experience of Victorian women throughout their life course also requires us to consider how to read the body within these intertwined individual and social experiences.

### *Embodiment Theory*

Embodiment theory, as formulated by anthropologist Thomas Csordas (1990), offers a framework to consider how our bodies are both objects of, and subjects in, our expressions of self, through the lens of cultural expectations and adherence to and deviance from social norms. In his words, studying embodiment "begins from the methodological postulate that the body is not an object to be studied in relation to culture, but is to be considered as the subject of culture, or in other words as the existential ground of culture" (Csordas 1990, 5). As we consider structural violence in the Victorian era, we need to weave in embodiment theory to uncover how the body reflects lived experiences in life, as the individual performed social expectations, and in death, as the body reveals the consequences of structural systems.

For bioarchaeological and biocultural studies, the body is central to analysis, but the addition of embodiment theory requires us to consider the larger constellation of the social and political lived experiences of the individuals we are examining. This means we need to consider the body as a transcript not only of direct experiences but also of indirect ones. The historical social subjects we examine, and the pathologies and traumas we can read from the skeletal body, need to be understood through a broader, intersectional lens that is informed by the cultural and environmental landscape. Employing embodiment theory, we can view the body as a site of information that is "simultaneously a subject and an object, meaningful and material, individual and social" (Mascia-Lees 2011, 1). In our analysis of the lived experiences of women in the Victorian era, the larger context of cultural and social systems, as explored through individual experiences, can inform and expand our understanding of how power and privilege worked to set the stage for social inequalities that have carried through to the present. For example, in the Victorian era, women who did not wear corsets were often referred to as "loose women," so called because of the perceived "looseness" of their morals as well as their uncorseted bodies. Moral judgments regarding a woman's sexual availability, drawn from Victorian codes for dress and behavior, shaped cultural understandings of the figure of the "fallen woman," who in her loss of social status also frequently lost the support of her family and/or employer as well as any means of economic sustenance. Under such circumstances, as we discuss in Chapter 4, women often had no recourse but to turn to sex work, suffering a further loss in status as well as risk to their health and wellbeing. In the case of the Victorian fallen woman, such structural violence may not necessarily have been direct or visible, as in bodily harm (although it might also take this path), but the consequence in the larger social arena was clear: fallen women did not conform to social norms and were shunned.

As these examples reveal, in any cultural context people are both shaped by and perform within a system of understanding that is comprised of individual, social, and political norms within that particular society. Within bioarchaeology, the body becomes a site to read definitions of "normality" and "deviance" through our understanding of cultural systems in place at the time, and in how we then read the presence or absence of certain health and pathological conditions. Embodiment and structural violence theory serve to inform our inquiries and shape the perspective that we engage to consider Victorian women throughout their life course. By relying on modern understandings of lived experience within this era, we must also include an examination of the intersections of ideology and embodiment in historical context in order to understand how Victorian women participated (and were policed) in the performance of social norms. In so doing, we strive to uncover the complexity of social experiences that can be read on the body, but need to be contextualized through the fabric of the social world in which the individual lived.

## *Intersectionality: Gender, Class, and Critical Race Theory*

> Intersectionality is a way of understanding and analyzing the complexity in the world, in people, and in human experiences. The events and conditions of social and political life and the self can seldom be understood as shaped by one factor. They are generally shaped by many factors in diverse and mutually influencing ways.
>
> (Collins and Bilge 2016, 1)

The term "intersectionality," coined by Kimberlé Crenshaw in 1989, enables us to see the ways in which multiple axes of privilege and oppression have historically operated, and continue to operate, to support cultural and societal structures of discrimination. Crenshaw's writings (1989, 2011), along with those of Derrick Bell (1995), Eduardo Bonilla-Silva (2015), Richard Delgado and Jean Stefancic (2001), and many others, been influential in shaping the field of critical race theory, which brings the analysis of race and racism to the fore in examining cultural, legal, economic, social, and many other aspects of human experience. In this project, we bring the insights of intersectionality and critical race theory to bear on our approach to studying Victorian female bodies in several ways. First, we argue that the skeletal evidence that has shaped the bioarchaeological record has skewed contemporary understandings of female bodily experience in the nineteenth century, because the majority of skeletons accessible for research today belong to poor women and women of color. Moreover, in studying cultural perceptions of women in Victorian England, we must acknowledge that this course of research focuses largely on white women, since very few people of color resided in England in the nineteenth century, and definitions of racial difference were further bound by assumptions about religion, culture, and ethnicity (Mitchell 1996; Steinbach 2017, 126). Regrettably, a comprehensive analysis of the bodies and lives of women of color in England and in the British colonies, particularly women of African, South Asian, and East Asian descent, lies beyond the scope of this book; however, this is a critical topic that merits further biocultural research to complement the existing scholarship in history and empire studies (Burton 1994; Burton 1998; Gerzina 2003; Salesa 2011). The paradox inherent in this analysis—that the assumptions regarding "the female body" in the Victorian era are implicitly classed and raced, that the dominant cultural narratives surrounding the Victorian woman are centered on white middle- and upper-class women, but are founded in research that has been limited to the bodies of poor and underprivileged white women and women of color—has inevitably structured our work. In what follows, we strive to remain attuned to the intersecting aspects of female identity and experience in Victorian England, while also recognizing the gaps and fissures in the historical and bioarchaeological record.

## The Victorian Era: An Overview

> The conviction is already not far from being universal, that the times are pregnant with change, and that the nineteenth century will be known to posterity as the era of one of the greatest revolutions of which history has preserved the remembrance, in the human mind, and in the whole constitution of human society.
>
> (Mill 1831, 169–170)

John Stuart Mill's (1831) remarks in "The Spirit of the Age," although published six years before the formal beginning of the Victorian era, aptly describe a population that conceived of its era as one of transformation. Writers then and since have attempted to sum up the "spirit of the age" using a variety of terms: the era has been characterized as everything from "an age of improvement" (Briggs 1959) to an "age of reform" (Woodward 1938; Brantlinger 1977). In the following section, we define some of the key features of the Victorian era, among them the important role played by industrialization and urbanization; imperialism and colonialism; scientific advancement; and new conceptions of gender and sexuality.

### *Characterizing the Victorian Era*

The Victorian era is named after Queen Victoria (1819–1901), whose accession to the throne on 20 June 1837 at the age of 18 marks the formal beginning of the period associated with her name (Altick 1973). She reigned for 63 years and seven months until her death on 22 January 1901—the longest reigning monarch in British history at the time. Victoria's long reign bridges historian Eric Hobsbawm's three epochs of the nineteenth century: the age of revolution (1789–1848), the age of capital (1848–1875), and the age of empire (1875–1914). The period was distinguished by dramatic economic growth alongside increasing disparities between the rich and the poor; the consolidation of power in the hands of the ruling classes in the face of protest at home and revolution abroad; and massive technological and industrial change. Significant demographic changes also occurred: the population of the United Kingdom almost doubled between 1800 and 1850, reaching 41.5 million in 1901 (Steinbach 2017, 3). Urbanization was a key factor in the transformation of the English landscape and everyday life in this era: London's population expanded from two million people in the 1840s to over six million by the end of the century, a transformation of the cityscape that was shared by cities in the industrial North. The urban population exceeded the rural population for the first time in the 1851 census, and remained so throughout the century. Patterns of migration from country to city led to overcrowding in urban districts, but the countryside was also in the process of being transformed as a result of the eighteenth-century enclosure movement (in which formerly common grazing lands were brought under the control of local landowners) and the shift from an agricultural to an industrial economy. The period was also marked by substantial imperial expansion: in India, for example, the Rebellion of 1857 (characterized by the British as the "Indian Mutiny") resulted in a formal shift in power from the East India Company to the British Crown, and in 1876, Victoria declared herself "Empress of India" (Cannadine 2001, 45). The "scramble for Africa" also took place over the course of the nineteenth century as explorers, scholars, and capitalists strove to exploit the resources of the African continent. The century concluded with the Anglo-Boer Wars (1880–1881 and 1899–1902, the latter now called the South African War), a decades-long struggle for control over the Transvaal and the Orange Free State in southern Africa. Arguably, Victorian England was structured in and through its status as an imperial nation: the displays of military might, the circulation and global exchange of goods, the networks of emigration and travel, the role of missionaries in perpetuating what came to be called Britain's "civilizing mission"—all symbolized the ways in which England understood itself to be the locus of imperial power across the globe (Said 1978, 1993; Burton 1998; Fischer-Tiné and Mann 2004; Logan 2010; Levine 2007).

### *Race, Colonialism, and Imperialism*

As the British Empire expanded across the globe during the nineteenth century, new cultures and peoples came under the lens of scientific analysis. Focusing on differences of language, culture, behavior, and physical appearance, Victorian scientists saw those outside of their insular, white, European communities as objects of study. As we discuss in Chapter 2, race became a central tenet in the movement to civilize, colonize, and otherwise distinguish white British citizens from all others. Victorian women were set against a racial hierarchy in which they were deemed less than their white male counterparts, but greater than all others. Victorian conceptions of normative citizenship were entrenched in the ideologies that constructed race as a biological concept, colonialism as central to the civilizing mission, and imperialism as a means to control and exploit the resources of foreign lands and peoples. The construction of femininity, civility, and norms for behavior must be understood within the larger social and ideological contexts of British imperialism and its effects on Victorian codes of morality and scientific inquiry. The imperial project in turn was bolstered by industrial and economic progress at home, which played a significant role in shaping the dynamics of class difference over the course of the nineteenth century.

## ***Class and the Industrial Revolution***

The Industrial Revolution, beginning in the eighteenth century, had a dramatic impact on the lived experience of Victorian women. Historians have debated the use of the term "revolution" to describe the societal transformations caused by the introduction of new technologies in agriculture, mining, and the industrial mass production of textiles, wrought iron, glass, and other Victorian commodities, as well as a variety of methods for creating greater efficiency through mechanization (Richards 1990). Scholars have suggested that the changes were more gradual rather than a sudden shift, and certainly they affected different sectors of society in different ways (Hopkins 2000; Steinbach 2017). Nonetheless, industrialization had a dramatic effect on the lives and health of Victorians, and occurred in concert with larger cultural changes. Class—whether defined in socioeconomic terms or through an individual's family background and upbringing—was a central factor in shaping Victorians' experience of industrialization (Williams 1976; Stedman Jones 1983). Under capitalism, for example, the factory owner benefited from the profits resulting from inducing employees to work long hours for low pay, while the factory workers (or "hands," as they were called in the period) were paid wages that were determined by management and the marketplace (Capuano 2015). Likewise, workers who took in "piecework," involving tasks such as sewing, tailoring, and other forms of work that could be undertaken at home, were paid by the item and subject to the whims of their employers with respect to their income and working hours. As we discuss in Chapter 3, the long hours, poor working conditions, and polluted skies that were characteristic of industrial capitalism and especially factory work led to significant legislative changes that in turn had a measurable effect on health. However, throughout the Victorian period, despite increased social mobility, greater leisure, and improvements to education and medicine, women across classes still suffered from both direct and indirect effects of an increasingly industrialized, urbanized environment.

### *Health and Illness*

The impact of industrialization on health and illness was dramatic, particularly for women and children and for those living in urban settings. Morbidity and mortality were increasing across classes as a result of both social and environmental factors. Victorian perceptions of mental health and the assumption that women were more susceptible to mental debility and illness (discussed in Chapters 2, 3, and 4) lent further support to the idea of the weak and less able female, and girded emergent systems of medical care and the science of difference. While one would think that with economic prosperity came improvements in health and greater access to care, this was not necessarily the case. From the smoke-clouded skies to exploitative labor conditions, from social expectations to the evolving field of biomedicine with its reliance on biological determinism and new ideas surrounding neurological and psychological etiologies of health, the Victorian period witnessed a decrease in overall wellness, especially for girls and women across the socioeconomic spectrum.

For the poor, children in particular suffered the largest consequences. The industrial revolution meant a dramatic increase in the number and severity of poorly nourished children, as a result of child labor in industrial factory settings, decline in exposure to sunshine, and lack of consistent access to food. The consequences of these social and environmental changes were children who were more susceptible to infection and disease, which can be measured in studies of reduced stature (height), and increases in morbidity (disease) and mortality (death) patterns for children during this era (all of which are discussed in more detail in Chapter 3).

For the elite, while it is true that the rich got richer, many also suffered from illness brought on by new models of care and a decline in physical exertion, as well as the adherence to certain moral codes and social expectations that had metabolic consequences. As with the poor, elite children, girls in particular, were likelier to suffer the consequences of ill health resulting from environmental and social changes. As we discuss in more detail in Chapter 3, the connections between wellness and the state of female reproductive capacity were seen as compromised by education, and often put at risk in the proper performance of beauty expectations. The increase in diagnoses of mental illness speaks to the newly developing science that was quick to label women as "hysterical"—a diagnosis that became all-encompassing, and offered further support for the ideology of the weakened and less able "civilized" female body. However, by the end of the nineteenth century, with changes in medical knowledge, the movement for women's rights (including greater access to higher education and professional opportunity), and dramatic changes in labor laws, regulatory measures, and other forms of legislation, health profiles improved for girls and women across classes.

### *Sexology and New Understandings of Gender and Sexuality*

The end of the nineteenth century witnessed a number of important legal, social, journalistic, and scientific interventions that affected the way gender and sexuality were seen in this era. Not only did challenges to the doctrine of separate spheres result in an expanded role for women in the professions; gender and sexuality also became part of the Victorian cultural conversation in new ways. In his pioneering work *The History of Sexuality* (of which the first volume was published in 1976), Michel Foucault argued that in contrast to popular perceptions of the Victorians as prudish and repressed—what he termed "the repressive hypothesis"—in fact discourses around sex and sexuality proliferated throughout this period, reverberating in new legislative and scientific categories delimiting gendered and sexual identities. Journalistic exposés like W. T. Stead's series of articles "The Maiden Tribute of Modern

Babylon," published in the *Pall Mall Gazette* in 1885, brought child prostitution, or what was then called the "white slave trade," into the public eye. Stead went undercover as a prospective client seeking to purchase a 13-year-old girl from her mother, in an effort to expose the sexual exploitation of girls and young women (Walkowitz 1992). Although child prostitution was rare, Stead's sensationalistic coverage helped pave the way for the passage of the Criminal Law Amendment Act, which raised the age of consent from 13 to 16, but also prompted other modes of legislating sexuality (Criminal Law Amendment Act 1885). Liberal MP Henry Labouchere's amendment to the Criminal Law Amendment Act made "gross indecency" between men a misdemeanor punishable by imprisonment; Oscar Wilde was prosecuted under the terms of this legislation in 1895. Several other scandals of the 1870s and 1880s were widely publicized, such as the 1870 case of Ernest Boulton and Frederick Park, who cross-dressed as women to attend theatres in London's West End, and the Cleveland Street scandal of 1889, which revealed to the public (or at least, published for the public's prurient interest) the fact that boys who worked delivering telegraphs for the London Post Office were also employed by a brothel on Cleveland Street that catered to aristocratic clients (Cohen 1996; Hindmarch-Watson 2012).

Meanwhile, British scientists in the emerging field of sexology drew on the scholarship of German sexologists, including Richard von Krafft-Ebing and Karl Heinrich Ulrichs, to articulate new frameworks for understanding and categorizing sexual desire (Bland 1995; Bland and Doan 1998a and 1998b). Ulrichs' (1864–1880) articulation of same-sex desire as natural, and his coinage of specific terminology ("urnings" for men who loved men, as well as terms for bisexual and intersex people), paved the way for a more expansive understanding of sexuality that is reflected in the work of the English writer and reformer Edward Carpenter, author of *Homogenic Love and Its Place in a Free Society* (1894) and *The Intermediate Sex* (1908). By contrast, Krafft-Ebing's *Psychopathia Sexualis* (1886) perpetuated a normative discourse around "normal" versus "deviant" sexual acts, and influenced a strain of sexology developed in the work of Havelock Ellis, whose *Studies in the Psychology of Sex* (1897–1910) coined the term "sexual inversion" to describe both male and female homosexuality. In the first volume of his study, co-authored with John Addington Symonds, Ellis defined sexual inversion as "sexual instinct turned by inborn constitutional abnormality towards persons of the same sex" (Ellis 1908, 96), and therefore challenged existing religious and medical discourses around homosexuality as a sin or a disease. Ellis's writings on lesbianism, however, perpetuated stereotypes of the "congenital female invert" as masculine and subject to a "hereditary taint" (Bland 1995, 263), and he maintained the biologically deterministic view that women's brains lay "in a sense [...] in their wombs" and that therefore motherhood was their true and natural purpose (Ellis, *Studies in the Psychology of Sex*, vol. 3, 253, cited in Bland 1995, 260). Ellis' writings, like other writings of the period that explicitly addressed homosexuality, were censored under Victorian obscenity laws, and difficult to obtain, making them read primarily by the scientific and medical community; yet gradually their work began to shift the cultural discourse around homosexuality and played an influential role in twentieth-century conversations about sexual acts, practices, and identities (Sedgwick 1985, 1990; Weeks 1985).

### *Science and Culture*

The convergence of scientific and cultural discourses in the work of the sexologists illuminates the complex ways in which the Victorians engaged with questions of gender, sexuality, and the body. In the following chapters, we address nineteenth-century discourses on science and sexuality, with particular attention to the period's focus on class, gender, and racial difference (Chapter 2); girlhood and adolescence (Chapter 3); marriage, pregnancy, and motherhood (Chapter 4); and menopause, aging, and death (Chapter 5). This focus on the life span of Victorian women enables us to address both the conventions associated with what Lyn Pykett terms "the proper feminine ideal" (Pykett 1992) as well as the ways in which Victorian women resisted the norms and conventions of the era. In our conclusion, we return to the relationship between science and culture, exploring possibilities for further research and inquiry into Victorian culture and its legacy today.

## Note

1 See the Human Rights Campaign's glossary at https://www.hrc.org/resources/glossary-of-terms and the American Psychological Association's "Definitions Related to Sexual Orientation and Gender Diversity in APA Documents," available here: https://www.apa.org/pi/lgbt/resources/sexuality-definitions.pdf.

## References

### *Primary Sources*

Carpenter, Edward. 1894. *Homogenic Love and Its Place in a Free Society*. Manchester: The Labour Press Society Limited.

Carpenter, Edward. 1908. *The Intermediate Sex: A Study of Some Transitional Types of Men and Women*. London: George Allen & Unwin Ltd.

Ellis, Havelock. 1908. *Studies in the Psychology of Sex*. 2nd ed. Philadelphia, PA: F. A. Davis and Co.

Krafft-Ebing, Richard von. 1886. *Psychopathia Sexualis*. 12th ed., 1903. Reprinted in *Sexology Uncensored: The Documents of Sexual Science*, edited by Lucy Bland and Laura Doan, 45–47, 77–90. Chicago, IL: University of Chicago Press, 1998.

Mill, John Stuart. 1831. "The Spirit of the Age." *Political Examiner*. Reprinted in *Romanticism: A Sourcebook*, 169–170, edited by Simon Bainbridge. Houndsmills, Basingstoke, Hampshire: Palgrave Macmillan, 2008.

Stead, W. T. 1885. "The Maiden Tribute of Modern Babylon." First published in the *Pall Mall Gazette* (6–10 July) and reprinted as *The Maiden Tribute of Modern Babylon* (*The Report of the "Pall Mall Gazette's" Secret Commission*) (London: Pall Mall Gazette).

Ulrichs, Karl Heinrich. 1864–1880. *The Riddle of "Man-Manly" Love: The Pioneering Work on Male Homosexuality*. Translated by Michael A. Lombardi-Nash, 1994. Buffalo, NY: Prometheus Books.

### *Secondary Sources*

Altick, Richard D. 1973. *Victorian People and Ideas: A Companion for the Reader of Victorian Literature*. New York: W. W. Norton and Company.

Bell, Derrick A. 1995. "Who's Afraid of Critical Race Theory?" *University of Illinois Law Review* 4: 893–910.

Bland, Lucy. 1995. *Banishing the Beast: English Feminism and Sexual Morality, 1885–1914*. London: Penguin, 2001.

Bland, Lucy, and Laura Doan, eds. 1998a. *Sexology in Culture: Labelling Bodies and Desires*. Chicago, IL: University of Chicago Press.

Bland, Lucy, and Laura Doan, eds. 1998b. *Sexology Uncensored: The Documents of Sexual Science*. Chicago, IL: University of Chicago Press.

Bonilla-Silva, Eduardo. 2015. "More than Prejudice: Restatement, Reflections, and New Directions in Critical Race Theory." *Sociology of Race and Ethnicity* 1 (1): 73–87.

Brantlinger, Patrick. 1977. *The Spirit of Reform: British Literature and Politics, 1832–1867*. Cambridge, MA: Harvard University Press.

Briggs, Asa. 1959. *The Age of Improvement, 1783–1867*. London: Longman.

Briggs, Asa. 1988. *Victorian Things*. London: Batsford.

Burton, Antoinette. 1998. *At the Heart of the Empire: Indians and the Colonial Encounter in Late-Victorian Britain*. Berkeley, CA: University of California Press.

Burton, Antoinette. 1994. *Burdens of History: British Feminists, Indian Women, and Imperial Culture, 1865–1915*. Chapel Hill: University of North Carolina Press.

Butler, Judith. 1990. *Gender Trouble: Feminism and the Subversion of Identity*. New York: Routledge.

Campbell, Frances. 2012. "Gilded Cages: The Trauma of Victorian Domesticity." Unpublished Division III Thesis. Amherst, MA: Hampshire College.

Cannadine, David. 2001. *Ornamentalism: How the British Saw Their Empire*. Oxford: Oxford University Press.

Capuano, Peter. 2015. *Changing Hands: Industry, Evolution, and the Reconfiguration of the Victorian Body*. Ann Arbor, MI: University of Michigan Press.

Cohen, William. 1996. *Sex Scandal: The Private Parts of Victorian Fiction*. Durham, NC: Duke University Press.

Collins, Patricia Hill, and Sirma Bilge. 2016. *Intersectionality*. Cambridge, England: John Wiley & Sons.

Collins Jr., James W., R. J. David, A. Handler, S. Wall, and S. Andes. 2004. "Very Low Birthweight in African American Infants: The Role of Maternal Exposure to Interpersonal Racial Discrimination." *American Journal of Public Health* 94 (12): 2132–2138.

Csordas, Thomas J. 1990. "Embodiment as a Paradigm for Anthropology." *Ethos* 18 (1): 5–47.

Crenshaw, Kimberlé. 1989. "Demarginalizing the Intersection of Race and Sex: A Black Feminist Critique of Antidiscrimination Doctrine, Feminist Theory and Antiracist Politics." *University of Chicago Legal Forum* 1 (8): 139–167.

Crenshaw, Kimberlé. 2011. "Twenty Years of Critical Race Theory: Looking Back to Move Forward." *Connecticut Law Review* 43 (5): 1253–1354.

Davis-Floyd, Robbie E., and Carolyn Fishel Sargent. 1997. *Childbirth and Authoritative Knowledge: Cross-Cultural Perspectives*. Berkeley, CA: University of California Press.

Delgado, Richard, and Stefancic, Jean. 2001; 2nd ed. 2012; 3rd ed. 2017. *Critical Race Theory: An Introduction*. New York: New York University Press.

Farmer, Paul, P. Bourgois, D. Fassin, L. Green, H. K. Heggenhougen, L. Kirmayer, L. Wacquant, and P. Farmer. 2004. "An Anthropology of Structural Violence." *Current Anthropology* 45 (3): 305–325.

Fausto-Sterling, Anne. 1993. "The Five Sexes: Why Male and Female Are Not Enough." *The Sciences* 33 (2): 20–25.

Fausto-Sterling, Anne. 2000. "The Five Sexes Revisited." *The Sciences* 40 (4): 18–23.

Fischer-Tiné, Harald, and Michael Mann, eds. 2004. *Colonialism as Civilizing Mission. Cultural Ideology in British India*. London: Anthem Press.

Foucault, Michel. 1976. *The History of Sexuality, Volume I*. Translated from the French by Robert Hurley, 1978. New York: Pantheon Books.

Galtung, Johan. 1969. "Violence, Peace, and Peace Research." *Journal of Peace Research* 6 (3): 167–191.

Galtung, Johan. 1990. "Cultural Violence." *Journal of Peace Research* 27 (3): 291–305.

Geller, Pamela. 2016. *The Bioarchaeology of Socio-Sexual Lives*. Switzerland: Springer International Publishing.

Gerzina, Gretchen Holbrook, ed. 2003. *Black Victorians/Black Victoriana*. New Brunswick, NJ: Rutgers University Press.

Giurgescu, C., B. L. McFarlin, J. Lomax, C. Craddock, and A. Albrecht. 2011. "Racial Discrimination and the Black–White Gap in Adverse Birth Outcomes: A Review." *Journal of Midwifery & Women's Health* 56 (4): 362–370.

Hindmarch-Watson, Katie. 2012. "Male Prostitution and the London GPO: Telegraph Boys' "Immorality" from Nationalization to the Cleveland Street Scandal." *Journal of British Studies* 51 (3): 594–617.

Hobsbawm, Eric. 1962. *The Age of Revolution: 1789–1848*. London: Weidenfeld and Nicolson.

Hobsbawm, Eric. 1975. *The Age of Capital, 1848–1875*. London: Weidenfeld and Nicolson.

Hobsbawm, Eric. 1987. *The Age of Empire: 1875–1914*. London: Weidenfeld and Nicolson.

Hopkins, Eric. 2000. *Industrialisation and Society 1830–1951*. London/New York: Routledge.

Jordan, Brigitte. 1993. *Birth in Four Cultures. A Crosscultural Investigation of Childbirth in Yucatan, Holland, Sweden and the United States*. Long Grove, IL: Waveland Press.

Joyner, Charles, W. 1999. *Shared Traditions: Southern History and Folk Culture*. Champaign, IL: University of Illinois Press.

Lepore, Jill. 2001. "Historians Who Love Too Much: Reflections on Microhistory and Biography." *The Journal of American History* 88 (1): 129–144.

Levine, Philippa. 2007. *The British Empire: Sunrise to Sunset*. Harlow, England/New York: Pearson Longman.

Lewis, Elizabeth. 2019. "What is Structural Violence? Anthropological Definitions and Examples." https://www.thoughtco.com/structural-violence-4174956. Accessed 8 December 2019.

Logan, Deborah A. 2010. *Harriet Martineau, Victorian Imperialism, and the Civilizing Mission*. Farnham, Surrey, England: Ashgate.

Loudon, Irvine. 1997. "Childbirth." In *Western Medicine: An Illustrated History*, edited by Irvine Loudon, 206–220. Oxford/New York: Oxford University Press.

Lu, M. C. and N. Halfon. 2003. "Racial and Ethnic Disparities in Birth Outcomes: A Life-Course Perspective." *Maternal and Child Health Journal* 7 (1): 13–30.

Marcus, Steven. 1966. *The Other Victorians: A Study of Sexuality and Pornography in Mid-Nineteenth Century England*. New York: Basic Books.

Martin, Deborah L. and Ryan P. Harrod. 2012. *The Bioarchaeology of Violence*. Gainesville, FL: University Press of Florida.

Mascia-Lees, Frances E. ed. 2011. *A Companion to the Anthropology of the Body and Embodiment* (Vol. 22). Hoboken, NJ: Wiley-Blackwell.

Mitchell, Sally. 1996. *Daily Life in Victorian England*. Westport, CT: Greenwood Press.

Murrell, Nancy L. 1996. "Stress, Self-Esteem, and Racism: Relationships with Low Birth Weight and Preterm Delivery in African American Women." *Journal of National Black Nurses' Association* 8 (1): 45–53.

Mustillo, S., N. Krieger, E. P. Gunderson, S. Sidney, H. McCreath, and C. I. Kiefe. 2004. "Self-Reported Experiences of Racial Discrimination and Black–White Differences in Preterm and Low-Birthweight Deliveries: The CARDIA Study." *American Journal of Public Health* 94 (12): 2125–2131.

Pykett, Lyn. 1992. *The "Improper Feminine": The Woman's Sensation Novel and the New Woman Writing*. Milton Park, Abingdon, Oxon/New York: Routledge.

Richards, Thomas. 1990. *The Commodity Culture of Victorian England: Advertising and Spectacle, 1851–1914*. Stanford, CA: Stanford University Press.

Said, Edward. 1978. *Orientalism*. New York: Pantheon Books.

Said, Edward. 1993. *Culture and Imperialism*. New York: Knopf.

Salesa, Damon Ieremia. 2011. *Racial Crossings: Race, Intermarriage, and the Victorian British Empire*. Oxford: Oxford University Press.

Sedgwick, Eve Kosofsky. 1985. *Between Men: English Literature and Male Homosocial Desire*. New York: Columbia University Press.

Sedgwick, Eve Kosofsky. 1990. *Epistemology of the Closet*. Berkeley, CA: University of California Press.

Stedman Jones, Gareth. 1983. *Languages of Class: Studies in English Working-Class History 1832–1982*. Cambridge: Cambridge University Press.

Steinbach, Susie L. 2012; 2nd ed. 2017. *Understanding the Victorians: Politics, Culture and Society in Nineteenth-Century Britain*. London/New York: Routledge.

Stone, Pamela K., 2009. "A History of Western Medicine, Labor, and Birth." In *Childbirth Across Cultures: Ideas and Practices of Pregnancy, Birth, and the Postpartum*, edited by Helaine Selin and Pamela K. Stone, 41–53. Dordrecht: Springer.

Stone, Pamela K., 2012. "Binding Women: Ethnology, Skeletal Deformations, and Violence Against Women." *International Journal of Paleopathology* 2 (2–3): 53–60.

Stone, Pamela K., 2016. "Biocultural Perspectives on Maternal Mortality and Obstetrical Death from the Past to the Present." *American Journal of Physical Anthropology* 159: 150–171.

Walkowitz, Judith. 1992. *City of Dreadful Delight: Narratives of Sexual Danger in Late-Victorian London*. Chicago, IL: University of Chicago Press.

Weeks, Jeffrey. 1985. *Sexuality and Its Discontents: Meanings, Myths, and Modern Sexualities*. London: Routledge and Kegan Paul.

Williams, Raymond. 1976. "Class." In *Keywords: A Vocabulary of Culture and Society*. New York: Oxford University Press.

Woodward, E. L. 1938; 2nd ed. 1962. *The Age of Reform, 1815–1870*. Oxford: Oxford University Press.

### *Online Resources*

Burnie, R. W. 1885. *The Criminal Law Amendment Act, 1885: With Introduction, Commentary, and Forms of Indictments*. London: Waterlow & Sons Limited. The British Library, shelfmark 6485.aaa.6. Available at: https://www.bl.uk/collection-items/the-criminal-law-amendment-act-1885. Accessed 23 March 2020.

# 2 Science, Evolution, and the Female Sex

## Introduction

The scientific pursuit to understand what makes us human became a driving force in the Victorian period. While still deeply steeped in religious belief systems based on the idea of a divine creator, Victorian scientists grappled with questions such as "What is at the root of human variations?" and "How did we get here?" As they pursued answers to these questions, they started to understand that "nature," "biology," and the "facts" of human similarity and difference were not reliant on supernatural forces, but rather the result of long histories of adaptation to different environments across the globe. While tensions did occur between the need to recognize, but not undermine, God's role in human creation, over the course of the nineteenth century scientific inquiry explored new ways to understand how humans evolved. These new methods also served to maintain the rigid cultural belief systems of the majority—white middle- and upper-class male scholars and practitioners of what was termed "natural science"—resulting in the justification of imperialist activities under the banner of the British Empire, and the colonization and study of cultural groups different from their own.

As the fields of biomedicine and science developed, human variation was seen through the lens of a dominant white and patriarchal narrative in which it was already pre-determined that European men, who were seen as the epitome of the civilized ideal, were the most evolved and therefore represented the normal body. All others, including white female bodies, were considered inferior. Even the eighteenth-century shift from a one-sex model to a two-sex model, described by historian Thomas Laqueur in his book *Making Sex: Body and Gender from the Greeks to Freud* (1990) and discussed at greater length below, was predicated on this narrative. These notions underlay how science framed the processes of evolution, underscoring Victorian scientists' own assumptions regarding what were assumed to be the criteria for an evolved and normal physical body: white, European, male, and God-fearing. This meant that these scientists' cultural conceptions of the meanings of the terms "normal" and "evolved" deeply influenced scientific and medical perspectives on human heredity, variation, and overall cognitive abilities.

This chapter examines how early Victorian scientists' understandings of human difference—including racial, sexual and gender difference, as well as differences in class, morality, and cognitive ability—were influenced by the cultural systems that they worked within. We investigate how Victorian moral and cultural codes influenced the ways in which empirical evidence was used to construct categories of human difference, including race and sex. We offer a brief examination of Victorian evolutionary thought and a working definition of biological determinism in order to underscore how the interpretation of empirical data was used to construct the superior white male as natural and evolved, against the perceived inferiority of the natural white female, and then all others, in a hierarchical model of racialized evolution. We then consider how the moral codes and the legal and social realities of the time reinforced the ways in which biological categories were seen. Victorian conceptions of gender, sexuality, and femininity both shaped and were shaped by biological determinism and scientific perspectives on human evolution, and Victorian women's lives were deeply influenced by long-held and powerfully normative ideologies of racial, sexual, and gender difference.

### *Darwin and Evolutionary Thought*

While direct evidence in the form of fossil remains of human ancestors would not be found until 1924, when Raymond Dart discovered the Taung Child (*Australopithecus africanus*) (Figure 2.1) in South Africa, Charles Darwin in his 1871 seminal text *The Descent of Man* speculated that one day fossils would be found connecting modern apes with modern humans via an ancient undiscovered common ancestor (Darwin 1871; White 2019). Although Darwin did not have explicit evidence that human evolution could be linked to other primates, his research, focusing on non-humans in the animal kingdom and culminating in his book *The Origin of Species* in 1859, addressed human origins as well as the origins of the other species he studied. Darwin is noted as the first scientist to articulate (in published form) a theory of evolution that was progressive, selective, and environmentally dependent).[1]

The most frequently cited example of Darwin's argument that variations within a species were tied to adaptations for survival comes from his study of finches, in which he hypothesized that adaptive strategies of the same species, separated by geographical distance, over multiple

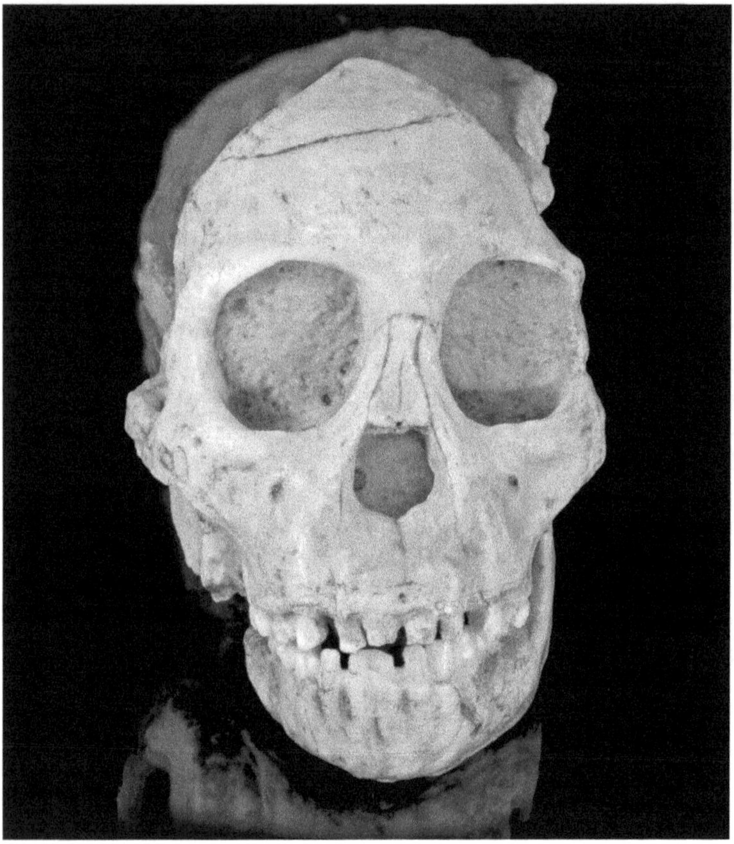

*Figure 2.1* Image of a cast of 2.1 million year old *Australopithecus africanus* specimen so-called Taung child, discovered in South Africa, 1924. Collection of the University of the Witwatersrand (Evolutionary Studies Institute), Johannesburg, South Africa. Sterkfontein cave, hominid fossil. Credit: Wikimedia Commons, Didier Descouens, CC BY-SA 3.0: https://commons.wikimedia.org/w/index.php?curid=29387940

generations would result in subtle as well as obvious changes in appearance and behaviors. This hypothesis formed the foundation of the concept of Natural Selection, in which adaptive changes allow an organism to survive and thrive in a particular environment, diverging from its original form (Figure 2.2). Darwin's observations of the physical and behavioral changes in the Galapagos finches helped him solidify his idea of natural selection, and ultimately his concept of "survival of the fittest," although this phrase

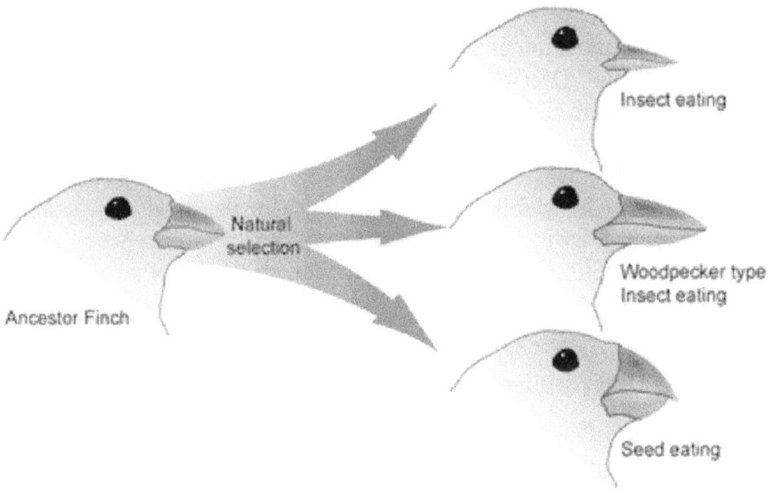


*Figure 2.2* Darwin's finches. Different variation of phenotype due to environment. National Human Genome Research Institute's Talking Glossary. http://geneed.nlm.nih.gov/topic_subtopic.php?tid=48

was actually coined by the sociologist Herbert Spencer, who was among the first to theorize the connections between Darwin's research and human evolution (Steinbach 2017). Spencer's writings popularized what came to be termed "Social Darwinism," which used evolutionary theory to justify imperial and colonial projects as well as to shape the evolving field of race science.

Like many Victorian scientists, Darwin believed that white Europeans represented an evolutionarily advanced human form. Theories of racial hierarchy and a progression from "primitive" to "civilized" societies shaped Darwin's understanding of white European culture as further along, evolutionarily speaking, as a result of having had more time to acquire the appropriate traits of civilization (Elliott 2003). Many of Darwin's contemporaries, including his cousin Sir Francis Galton, who coined the term "eugenics" in 1883, used his work as a scientific proof of evolution's role in establishing race as a biological category, fueling perceptions of difference and racial hierarchy as well as practices of economic exploitation, colonization, and enslavement.

Darwin's views on human variation extended to his views on sex differences, which were also shaped by the conventional perceptions of his time. Darwin argued that the result of sexual selection was that man was "more courageous, pugnacious and energetic than woman [with] a more inventive genius" (Darwin 1871, 316). He further claimed that sex differences could be identified in the size of the male and female brain: "His brain is absolutely larger [...] the formation of her skull is said to be intermediate between the child and the man" (Darwin 1871, 317). Darwin's belief that males evolve in order to meet the chosen criteria of strength and power supported by the rigid Victorian cultural systems of the nineteenth century was crucial in underscoring the theory of a clear differentiation between the sexes, and thus provided an alleged biological basis for the physical and social superiority of men. Darwin's work on human variation was entrenched in the biological determinism that, in turn, structured ideologies of gender, class, and race in the Victorian period.

## Biological Determinism

> [The] claim that natural and intrinsic inequalities between individual human beings at birth are determinative of eventual differences in their status, wealth, and power [...] is the defining property of biological determinism.
>
> (Lewontin 1983, 153)

The concept of biological determinism, which developed from eighteenth- and nineteenth-century understandings of heredity, argues that all aspects of a person, from physical characteristics, to mental/cognitive abilities, to behaviors, are hardwired at conception, and virtually unable to be changed. Working within biologically deterministic theories of human physiology, nineteenth-century scientists interested in quantifying human differences relied on anthropometry, or the study of measurements of proportion and size of the physical (anatomical) features of the human body. Some of these anthropometric measures included cranial capacity, height, weight, as well as bumps on the head (integral to phrenology, described below), height of cheek bones, size of the brow ridge, and size and shape of the nose. Often these measures were then associated with perceived mental and personality traits, and purported to show how anatomical characteristics can reveal an individual's degree of intelligence and underlying moral and behavioral characteristics.

A striking example of how anthropometry was used to make the case for biological determinism can be seen in the work of Cesare Lombroso, who is known as the "father of modern criminology" (Walsh and Ellis 2006). Lombroso believed in the theory of the "born criminal," and studied the insane, as well as known criminals, to amass a catalogue of physical features that he saw as the "hallmarks" of a criminal. Lombroso's belief system and his efforts to quantify criminal traits arose from Ernst Haeckel's biogenetic law (1866), which stated that ontogeny (individual development) recapitulates phylogeny (evolutionary development of the species). This theory prompted Lombroso's focus on the idea that "criminals are born criminal and that they are evolutionary 'throwbacks' to an earlier form of life" (Walsh and Ellis 2006, 60).

The now-discredited science of phrenology—the practice of reading the size and shape of bumps on the skull and linking them to the "organs" or faculties associated with psychological and behavioral qualities—was first developed in the late eighteenth century by the Austrian physician Franz Joseph Gall (Figure 2.3).

Although Gall used little evidence in developing his theory of the correlation between skull shape and psychological characteristics, it nonetheless

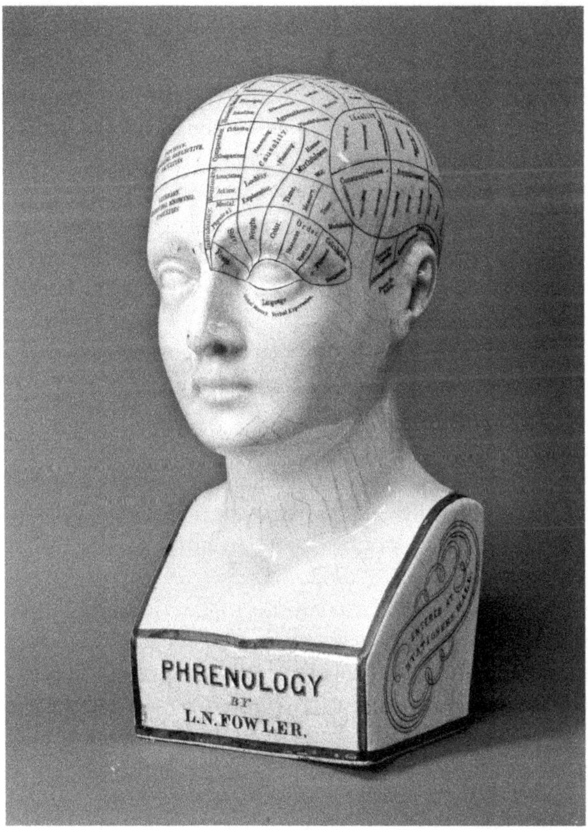


*Figure 2.3* "Phrenology," a ceramic head. Credit: Wellcome Collection: https://wellcomecollection.org/works/wz7p6v6b

gained popularity in Britain and the United States as well as in Europe in the early decades of the nineteenth century. References to phrenology can be found throughout Victorian literature: in *Jane Eyre*, for example, the protagonist describes her teacher Miss Temple as having "a considerable organ of veneration," and skeptically evaluates her employer Mr. Rochester as possessing "a solid enough mass of intellectual organs, but an abrupt deficiency where the suave sign of benevolence should have risen" (Brontë 1847; Dames 2001). Gall's writings, and those of his contemporaries including Johann Gaspar Spurzheim and George Combe, were influential in shaping the theories espoused by Lombroso and other studies of personality, character, and psychology prior to the rise of psychoanalysis in the later Victorian period (Gilman 1985; Walsh and Ellis 2006).

Lombroso was not the only theorist to consider the role of biology as deterministic not only to physical traits but to behavioral ones as well. Anthropologists of the times were also assessing cultures across the globe with this same idea. For example, in 1882 Dr. George Engelmann published the first edition of his text *Labor Among Primitive Peoples*, detailing his many years of work around the globe, in which he sought to conduct "a comparison of the crude methods of Primitive Peoples and Peoples of former civilizations with the teachings of scientific obstetrics of to-day [sic]" (Engelmann 1882, xv). His work examines multiple aspects of reproduction, including abortion, labor and birth, birthing positions, and the interactions of the parturient with family and midwives/birth attendants, as well as in their own lived experiences. Engelmann reflects on the differences between those who are "nearer to civilization" versus "those who live in a natural state," concluding that with "any deviation from these natural conditions, trouble results" in childbirth (Engelmann 1882, 8). The idea that more "civilized" females were at higher risk for childbirth complications and death aligned well with the Victorian conception of the evolved female body as weaker and compromised by her reproductive capacities, yet also "elevated" above the "barbarous" state of being driven by passion rather than reason (Laqueur 1990, 189).

Given the biologically deterministic frameworks of the Victorian period, the ideologies and behaviors surrounding the concept of "civilization" were seen as the hallmark of a more highly evolved society. As a result, cultural groups that were radically different from white Europeans (as Engelmann's work aimed to explore) were seen as less evolved. It was this ideology of biological—hence cultural and racial—difference that gave support to British colonial enterprises, as the British were able to claim their superiority over other culturally different groups in the name of God and civilization. Moreover, in perpetuating the ideology of the "civilizing mission," Victorian imperialists strove to underscore their assumed moral superiority in relation to other colonial powers such as the French, the Dutch, and the Belgians—the latter of whom were represented as especially rapacious and brutal in their efforts to conquer and exploit the riches of colonized lands in Africa and Asia (Davin 1978; Said 1993; Fischer-Tiné and Mann 2004; Logan 2010).

### *The Construction of Racial Difference*

As the British Empire expanded, the need to assert superiority over colonized peoples coalesced in the development of nineteenth-century theories of racial, cultural, and ethnic difference. Race became a central tenet differentiating people into categories that were perceived as biologically real. For the Victorian natural scientist, human racial categories and racial differences were also a central focus, as visible physical differences were seen as in need of categorization. Efforts to classify individuals into distinct categories based on assumed racial, ethnic, and cultural differences had long-lasting repercussions, informing the foundations of the eugenicist theories constructed by Francis Galton in the late nineteenth century, which were ultimately appropriated for political and other purposes.

Victorian race science was structured by a biologically deterministic ethos, which relied heavily on anatomy, morphology, and typology, to develop an understanding of human difference, and to "support the idea that certain human groups were intrinsically inferior to others" (Stepan 1982, ix). The binary concepts of "civilized" and "savage," along with associated conceptions of moral character and closeness or distance from God, were seen as central modes through which biology could be categorized. In the construction of human racial difference, these conceptual distinctions helped early scientists to define race as both a product of the physical body and a psychological experience. Likewise, the perceived difference between the sexes rested on the foundation of biologically determined, but actually culturally constructed, distinctions between male and female.

### *The Construction of Sex and Gender Difference*

As noted, nineteenth-century scientific and medical opinion viewed female bodies as unequal to their male counterparts. Since biology was seen as absolute and inescapable, the medical story was clear: differences were "designed by nature as a necessary basis to ensure the social order between men, women, and the family" (Pockles, as cited by Schiebinger 1986, 69). With science proving that "natural inequalities" existed (Schiebinger 1993), this framework also supported the contention that "white women ranked below European men in scales of both ontogeny and phylogeny"

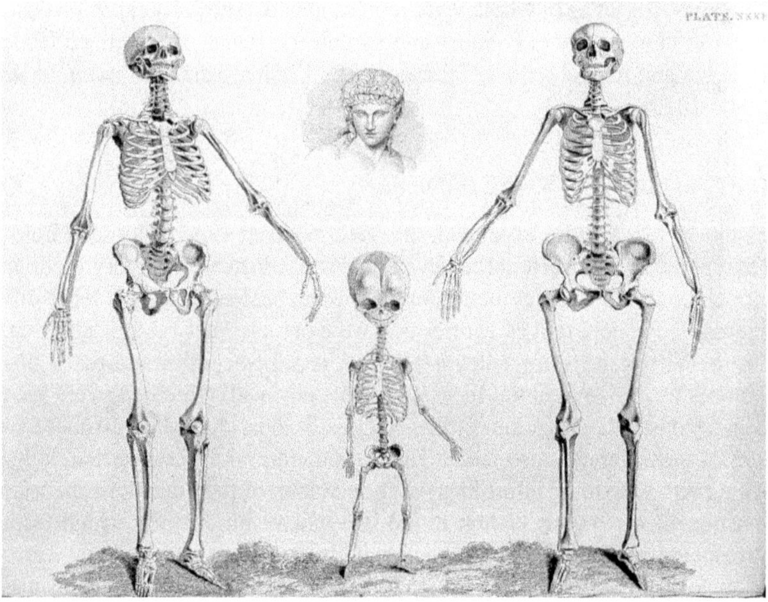


*Figure 2.4* *The Anatomy of the Bones*, 1829. Credit: Wellcome Collection: https://wellcomeimages.org/indexplus/image/L0028782.html

(Schiebinger 1986, 63). While all women were considered inferior to white men, white female bodies were still seen as evolutionarily superior to all other non-white identified female bodies who ranked further down the evolutionary chain. Such erroneous assessments embedded in Victorian conceptions of gender and race led to the purportedly normal, universal female body being labeled as child-like, weak, fragile, and white (Figure 2.4).

As Thomas Laqueur argues in *Making Sex: The Body and Gender from the Greeks to Freud*, prior to the eighteenth century, the predominant view centered on a one-sex model which held that the female body was the inverse of the male. In the Galenic view (based on the writings of the ancient Greek physician Galen in the second century A.D. and theories of the bodily fluids or "humors"), "women were essentially men in whom a lack of vital heat—of perfection—had resulted in the retention, inside, of structures that in the male are visible without" (Laqueur 1990, 4). In the seventeenth and eighteenth centuries, scientists began to evolve what is now called the two-sex model, in which male and female physiology was seen as fundamentally distinct:

> The dominant, though by no means universal, view since the eighteenth century has been that there are two stable, incommensurable, opposite sexes and that the political, economic, and cultural lives of men and women, their gender roles, are somehow based on these 'facts.' Biology—the stable, ahistorical, sexed body—is understood to be the epistemic foundation for prescriptive claims about the social order.
>
> (Laqueur 1990, 6)

This model existed against a backdrop of moral codes in which anatomical differences were stressed and biological and behavioral differences were seen as locked in, stemming from the "nerves, flesh, and bone" (Harvey 2002, 901).

Over the last two centuries, anthropology and medicine have continued to use the same criteria to narrowly define the differences between male and female bodies (Cannon-Mohammed 2018). In the Victorian period in particular, such strategies were used to reject or critique the possibility of political change: as one text claimed, "What was decided among the prehistoric Protozoa cannot be annulled by an act of Parliament" (Geddes and Thompson 1889, 266, cited in Laqueur 1990). These scientifically rendered facts about human difference, as rooted in biology, allow for the objectification of the female body, and in particular the non-white female body, making it a site of colonial enterprise and inquiry.

## Female Bodies as Subjects of Victorian Science

Such culturally constructed ideas of race and sex, supported through scientific studies, meant that early anatomists embraced evolutionary explanations which proposed "that differences between male and female bodies were so vast that women's development had been arrested at a lower stage of evolution" (Schiebinger 1986, 63). These arguments were reinforced by females' generally smaller stature, crania, ribs and feet, their gracile mandibles, and the fact that they generally stopped growing by age fourteen (Schiebinger 1986). Victorian scientists then translated these physical traits into their attempts to categorize women by their perceived behaviors. The scientific logic was that since female bodies were physically more childlike, women's behaviors and intellects were more childlike as well (Schiebinger 1986). Medical understanding now had (or believed it had) direct biological support to prove that women's bodies were unequal to those of their male counterparts (Harvey 2002). Of course, the most distinguishing characteristic that set females apart from males was their ability to gestate and bear children. In biological terms, biology shaped sex, so the focus of sex differences was to be highlighted through a focus on reproduction, the pelvis (discussed in more detail in subsequent chapters), and race.

Human variation and the construction of the "normal" female body were girded by the developing Victorian discourse around the science of human reproduction and racial differences. Placing white female bodies within a political field of power and privilege, and highlighting their normative status with respect to other bodies, set the white female apart from all others. Deviance from this constructed cultural norm resulted in non-white female bodies becoming sites of analysis and inquiry, while also serving to protect the normal white female body from study.

### *Intersecting Ideologies of Racial and Sexual Difference: The "Hottentot Venus"*

The rise in status of science, and the focus on the early evolutionary theory that different races evolved from different ancestors, known as the polygenetic model of human difference, enabled science to unabashedly colonize and dissect non-white bodies. The nineteenth-century study and display of the sexualized black female became a mode by which Victorians could publicly distinguish the so-called "primitive" from the "civilized" (white) female form. Victorian scientific discourse aligned with imperial expansion and colonial trade to assure that white European-born male scientists could prosper in the pursuit of colonizing non-white bodies as well.

An important example of the extreme ways Victorian men of science explored both racial and sex differences in non-white female bodies in the name of scientific inquiry comes from the case of Sara Baartman (also known as Saartjie, Sartjee, and Sarah Bartmann), a young woman taken from Cape Colony in South Africa and brought to England in 1810 to be exhibited as an example of "that most wonderful phenomenon of nature, the Hottentot Venus: the only one ever exhibited in Europe" (Figure 2.5). For scientists, and public voyeurs of the time, she represented the distinguishing features of the "lowest rung on the great chain of being" and was seen as the "central nineteenth-century icon for sexual difference between the European and the black" (Gilman 1985, 212). While in life she was viewed as exotic as well as erotic, her death allowed for additional insults by the colonial race science of the Victorian period (Crais and Scully 2009).

After her untimely death, Sara Baartman's body was dissected with "two intentions: to compare a female of the 'lowest' human species with the highest ape (the orangutan) and describe the anomalies of the Hottentot's 'organ of generation'" (Gilman 1985, 213). The scientific effort to use Baartman's body as evidence for theories of atavism and racial progress, as well as for phrenological analysis, operated through a fetishistic colonial discourse based

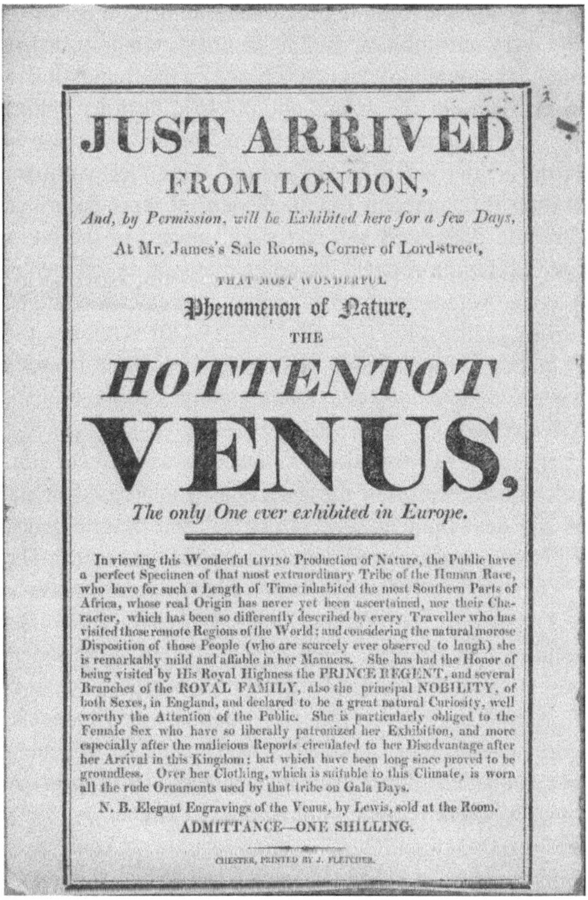


*Figure 2.5* Advertisement for the exhibition of the Hottentot Venus, c. 1810. Credit: Wellcome Collection: https://wellcomecollection.org/works/svbbasrz

on an explicit "articulation of the visual forms of corporeal racial/sexual difference" (Netto 2005, 151–152). This work exemplifies the larger systemic approach to codifying scientific racism, in which Victorian science used black bodies to cement assumptions of "biological" difference as deviance.

### ***Victorian Bodies and Codes: Hysteria***

While Sara Baartman's body was displayed and dissected, the bodies of white women were covered and protected. However, both white and non-white women were subjected to evolving conceptions of gendered physiological deviance that were grounded in biologically deterministic theories of difference. Indeed, the very terminology used to describe certain disorders associated with (though not limited to) women is based on the foundation of biological determinism. Hysteria, the mental and physical disorder almost exclusively associated with women in the nineteenth century, is a case in point. The word "hysteria" derives from "hysteron," the Greek word for uterus. As early as 1900 B.C., ancient Egyptian medical texts described an organ that had become dislocated and had risen upward in the body. Subsequently, ancient Greek philosophers including Plato attributed mental disorders in women to the "wandering womb," whose movements could be traced to a lack of sexual gratification (Micale 1995, 19–20). Although the concept of a literally mobile uterus faded through lack of evidence, hysteria in its classical form was fundamentally defined through its association with the female reproductive system.

A wide range of etiological explanations followed in subsequent centuries, including the characterization of the hysterical woman as demonically possessed and the development of neurological and psychological explanations for the symptoms associated with hysteria (Micale 1995). The constitutive feature of hysteria—its characterization as a feminine disease—remained, however.[2] Perhaps the most famous nineteenth-century theorists of hysteria were the French neurologist Jean-Martin Charcot, who undertook a series of photographic and analytical studies of hysterical women at the Salpêtrière in Paris; and Sigmund Freud, who studied with Charcot in the 1880s and who later developed his approach to psychoanalytic treatment through his case studies of patients like Bertha Pappenheim, who appears as "Anna O" in *Studies in Hysteria* (co-authored with Josef Breuer in 1895), and Ida Bauer, whom Freud renamed "Dora" in "Fragment of an Analysis of a Case of Hysteria" (Showalter 1985, 155–160). As Elaine Showalter notes in her pioneering study *The Female Malady: Women, Madness, and English Culture, 1830–1980*, in its early years psychoanalysis offered an alternative to the constricting assumptions of biological determinism and what she terms "Darwinian psychiatry" (Showalter 1985, 105–106), epitomized by the work of Henry Maudsley, Cesare Lombroso, and others. However, the British medical establishment was hesitant to accept the main feature of psychoanalysis—the "talking cure"—and instead privileged other forms of treatment, including institutionalization, surgical interventions, and other forms of controlling the female body in order to regulate the female mind.

The Victorian period marks a turning point in the gendering of mental illness. By the mid-nineteenth century, women outnumbered men in public asylums and—importantly—were thought "to be more vulnerable to insanity than men, to experience it in specifically feminine ways, and to be differently affected by it in the conduct of their lives" (Showalter 1985, 52, 7). Mental illness was also perceived as more likely to affect highly civilized, indeed "over-civilized," populations—especially in industrialized nations, and especially white women of the middle and upper classes (Briggs 2000). Indeed, class was a central component in determining how a woman with mental illness would be treated in the Victorian era. The passage of the Lunacy Act of 1845 required county governments to construct and manage public lunatic asylums, and to keep records regarding the treatment of patients; prior to this point, people suffering from mental illness who could not afford a private asylum or the fees associated with a registered hospital would be likely to end up in the workhouse or in prison. The figure of the "madwoman in the attic," who occupied a central role in early Victorian fiction, gave way to the institutionalized woman of the later nineteenth century.

In summary, throughout the Victorian period and into the twentieth century, doctors and psychiatrists were convinced that women were more likely to experience mental illness because their reproductive systems rendered them less able to control their emotions, mental states, and sexual and physical responses. Diseases of the mind, especially hysteria and its varied forms, were diseases of the body, and the female body itself must be brought under control in order for women to take up their proper place in society.

## Sexuality and Social Ideals

As the example of hysteria demonstrates, women's bodies were at the center not only of medical and scientific debates in the Victorian period, but also vital to cultural and social discourses around the relationship between femininity and masculinity and the debates over what was termed "the woman question" in the nineteenth century (Helsinger et al. 1983). In what follows, we explore the social ideals that underpinned Victorian ideologies of gender and sexual difference, paying particular attention to the moral codes that governed women's behavior. We examine the changing legal status of women in the nineteenth century, and explore the shift involved in women's struggle for university education and the battle for entry into the medical profession. Lastly, we consider how women resisted Victorian norms of marriage and motherhood: in literature and popular culture, the figures of the spinster, the "odd woman," and the New Woman offered a range of new social roles and opportunities as the century came to a close.

### *Ideologies of Femininity*

As scholars have argued, relationships between men and women in Victorian England were shaped by an ideology of separate and gendered spheres—which, notably, was more perception than reality: a culturally constructed and largely illusory model that was unobtainable for (or unwanted by) most women. Nonetheless, the separate spheres ideology had a dramatic influence over cultural and societal norms throughout the period. As a result, Victorian society was guided by strict codes of gender difference that shaped behavior and delineated identities, particularly for the white middle and upper classes. Working-class women were likewise guided by a commitment to respectability that also governed their behavior in keeping with class and gender norms. In what follows, we address the relationship between class and gender in shaping ideologies of femininity in the Victorian era, focusing on the similarities and differences across class and economic lines.

Prior to the Industrial Revolution, middle-class women and men worked alongside one another in agricultural settings within a model based on the understanding that members of a family (or equivalent social structure) were partners in a shared economic enterprise (Davidoff and Hall 1987). However, with the rise of industrial capitalism, and the emergence of an economic system predicated on increased specialization and professionalization that separated men's labor from the enterprise of the household, women—especially, but not only, middle-class women—were increasingly encouraged to associate themselves with the so-called private sphere of domesticity (Langland 1995). Men employed in the public realm in jobs ranging from factories and offices to professional settings as doctors, lawyers, clergymen, and educators were expected to display the characteristics associated with Victorian masculinity—stoicism, the "stiff upper lip," restraint and strength—and to be the primary breadwinners for their families (Steinbach 2017). Women, by contrast, were trained to embody the characteristics of "the angel in the house" (the name of a popular poem by Coventry Patmore, which we discuss further in Chapter 3): to be keepers of the hearth, guardians of morality, efficient domestic managers, and loving wives and mothers. Women took primary responsibility for bearing, rearing, and educating children, and were also expected to minister to the needs of their husbands. However, the realities of class and economic change over the course of the century meant that women of all but the most wealthy classes worked both within and outside the home, in forms of labor that were both paid (factory and shop work, dressmaking, plain sewing, and piecework, as well as in professional careers as nurses, governesses, and teachers) and unpaid (a wide variety of tasks associated with the maintenance of the home, thought to be their unique purview). Indeed, the prevalence of women in the teaching and caretaking professions throughout this period speaks to the influence of the separate spheres ideology, which characterized women as nurturing, morally superior, and wise (Copelman 1996; Judd 1998; Hallam 2000; Hawkins 2010).

A feminine ideal based on this gendered ideology emerges in both fiction and non-fiction in this period. In novels ranging from Charles Dickens' *Oliver Twist* (1837) to George Eliot's *The Mill on the Floss* (1860), and in other contexts ranging from poetry and song to painting and illustration, the ideal woman was beautiful, fair-skinned and fair-haired, decorous, submissive, and often child-like. The depiction of the fragile (and implicitly white) female body as the norm, indeed the ideal representation of Victorian womanhood, underpins the scientific discourses discussed previously, which serve to codify and reinforce racial and class distinctions throughout the century.

Needless to say, there were always exceptions to this normative middle-class ideology of femininity. Working-class women and women of color were, on the one hand, expected to heed the hegemony of the period's gender norms, but on the other they were also expected to be physically strong in order to work as domestic servants, farm laborers, and factory workers. These ideological norms ignore the presence of much more varied gender identities and sexual practices. For example, heteronormative understandings of love and marriage belie the realities of gay, lesbian, bisexual, and what we would now call queer and trans identities in the Victorian era (Vicinus 2004; Marcus 2007).

### *Moral Codes and Gender Roles*

As Michel Foucault's pioneering work *The History of Sexuality* argues, the nineteenth century marked a proliferation in discourses around sexuality, and the Victorian investment in classification and categorization meant that this was the era in which sexual identities and norms were delimited and codified. As a result, throughout the Victorian period, sexuality was subject to a set of binary distinctions associated with the sexual double standard. Such distinctions led to complex negotiations around gender, sexuality, and morality. Men were seen as naturally sexual beings, and were thought likely to gain sexual experience before marriage, either through relationships with unmarried women (in some cases, domestic servants in their families' employ), or through recourse to prostitutes (Steinbach 2017). Women, by contrast, were imagined to be asexual beings, more concerned with moral and spiritual purity than with sexual desire and fulfillment.

Emblematic of the links between purity, womanhood, and nationalism, the quote "Lie back and think of England," so often misattributed to Queen Victoria, is more stereotype than reality. However, women were expected to be (or at least to appear) passionless and pure, and virginal both in their marriage bed and beyond. In the words of historian Barbara Welter, the "cult of true womanhood" espoused in American popular magazines from 1820 to 1860 emphasized the "four cardinal virtues": "piety, purity, submissiveness and domesticity" (Welter 1976, 21). British women were similarly expected to maintain chastity and virginity until marriage, and to submit to their husbands' wishes regarding the timing, frequency, and occurrence of sexual intercourse. Scholarship into the lives and writings of Victorian women—Queen Victoria among them—has gone a long way toward dispelling the stereotype of women as asexual, passionless, and chaste; but the prevailing moral codes were nonetheless influential in shaping understandings of gender and sexuality throughout this period (Munich 1996; Homans and Munich 1997).

Victorian moral codes were bound up in larger legal and social realities that disenfranchised all women, some more than others. The patriarchal structure of Victorian society meant that women were passed from the supervision of their fathers to that of their husbands; unmarried daughters were expected to remain at home and serve as caretakers for their parents and siblings. The system of coverture—in which a woman was considered *feme sole* until her marriage, when she became *feme covert*—resulted in women's loss of independent legal status. As Sir William Blackstone famously put it in his *Commentaries on the Laws of England* (1765):

> By marriage, the husband and wife are one person in law; that is, the very being and legal existence of the woman is suspended during the marriage, or at least is incorporated and consolidated into that of the husband: under whose wing, protection, and *cover*, she performs everything.
>
> (Blackstone 1765)

Until 1870, a woman's personal property became her husband's upon marriage, and she could not retain any earnings for her own use until the passage, between 1870 and 1884, of a series of laws addressing married women's property (this legislation is discussed at greater length in Chapter 4). Married women could not enter into legal contracts, could not sue or be sued, were not liable for their own debts, and were physically and morally considered subject to their husbands' absolute will and power. In her 1854 text *A Brief Summary, in Plain Language, of the Most Important Laws Concerning Women*, feminist Barbara Leigh Smith framed the situation thus: "A woman's body belongs to her husband: she is in his custody, and he can enforce his right by a writ of *habeas corpus*" (Smith 1854, 4). Under these conditions, marital rape did not exist, and women had little legal recourse in cases of domestic abuse (Mill 1869).

The structural discrimination against women embedded in the Victorian legal system extended to women's struggle for citizenship, embodied by the women's suffrage movement from the 1860s to the passage of the Representation of the People Acts of 1918 and 1928, which granted the vote to women over thirty and to women over twenty-one, respectively. Many Victorian feminists and suffrage activists based their call for equal rights for women on the effort to combat the sexual double standard that structured women's legal, social, economic, and physical lived experience. A case in point is the effort to repeal the Contagious Diseases Acts (passed in 1864 and 1866, with amendments in 1868 and 1869, and repealed in 1886), a movement led by feminist reformer Josephine Butler in the 1870s and 1880s.

The Contagious Diseases Acts were an effort to control the spread of venereal disease in military garrisons and port towns by legislating control over the bodies of sex workers: women could be apprehended merely on suspicion of prostitution, and were subject to placement in "lock hospitals" as well as compulsory examination and treatment. It was not lost on feminists that men were not subject to similar action, and reformers framed their arguments based on the infringement of women's civil rights and what was termed the "instrumental violation" of the forced medical examination using the newly available speculum (Walkowitz 1980; Jordan 2007; Sanders 2015). The repeal effort was ultimately successful, and became a testament to the power of women's ability to organize and advocate for equal treatment under the law. Nonetheless, as we discuss in Chapter 4, Victorian sex workers were still subject to discrimination throughout the century, and women who were sexually active outside of marriage were stigmatized as "fallen women" (Anderson 1993) (Figure 2.6).

The debate over the Contagious Diseases Acts, and the activism associated with the rise of feminist reform efforts in a variety of arenas, symbolized the importance of the call for an end to the sexual double standard. Prominent Victorian feminists drew clear connections between morality and legal freedom: Millicent Garrett Fawcett, the leader of the constitutional suffrage movement, called for a "higher moral standard in the community at large, and especially a higher moral standard among men," and Josephine Butler saw the vote as the way to obtain moral "justice" in striving for "an equal code of morality, *one standard* for men and for women alike, equal laws based upon an equal standard" (Fawcett, cited in Rubinstein 1991, 92; Butler, cited in Jordan 2007, 118).

### *Acts of Resistance: Women and the Medical Profession*

Women's activist efforts in the nineteenth century extended to the realms of education and the professions, particularly the medical profession. Prior

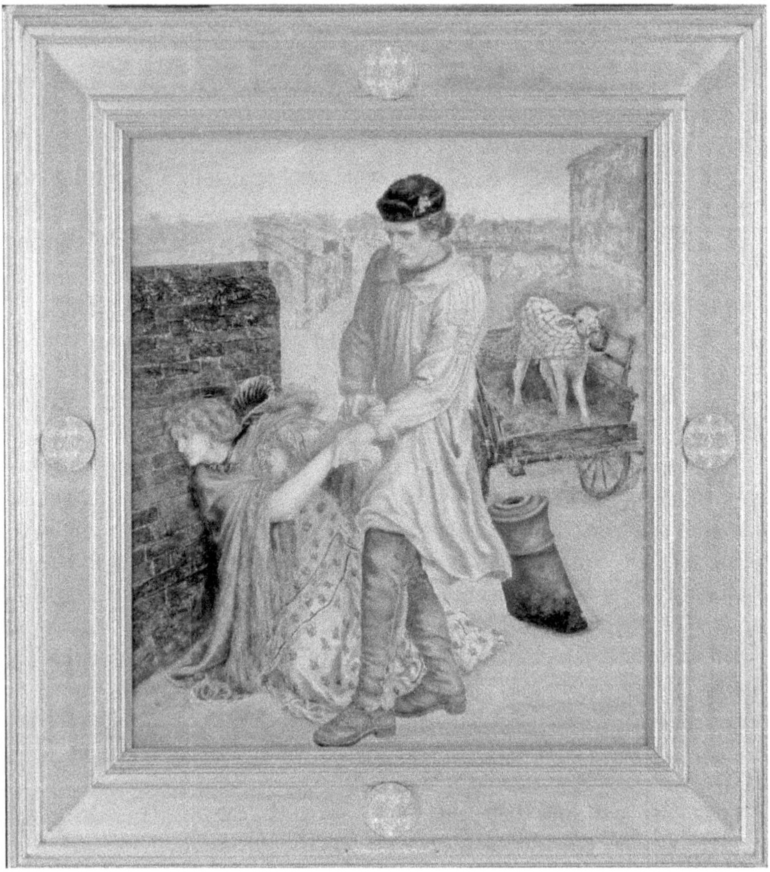

*Figure 2.6* Dante Gabriel Rossetti, *Found.* Designed 1853; begun 1859 (unfinished). Oil on canvas. Delaware Art Museum, Samuel and Mary R. Bancroft Memorial, 1935. Object number 1935–27.

to the 1860s, women were barred from entry to medical schools and could not obtain degrees to practice medicine. Yet women longed for the opportunity to seek medical treatment from licensed female physicians. Josephine Butler lamented, "How would any modest man endure to put himself in the hands of a woman medically as women have to put themselves into the hands of men? And are women less modest than men?" Having consulted with Elizabeth Garrett, the first woman licensed to practice medicine in Britain, Butler observed, "I must say of her that I gained more from her than from any other doctor [...] because I was able to tell her so much more than

I ever could or would tell to any man" (Josephine Butler to Albert Rutson, 22 February 1868; cited in Petrie, *A Singular Iniquity*, 65–66). Yet societal prejudices against women serving as medical practitioners ran deep, and women had to fight a lengthy battle to gain access to medical training and certification.

Women had been health practitioners for centuries, whether serving as midwives or in offering daily care to family and community members through well-known herbs, tinctures, home remedies and other healing practices, and catching babies. Domestic manuals such as Isabella Beeton's famous text *Mrs. Beeton's Book of Household Management* (first published in 1861) offered guidance on everything from practical housekeeping tips to chapters on "Invalid Cookery" and "The Rearing and Management of Children, and Diseases of Infancy and Childhood." The ideological association between women, domesticity, and caretaking meant that when middle-class women sought professional training in the mid-nineteenth century, they began by entering fields that had historically been gendered feminine; most prominent amongst these was the field of nursing. In her 1852 essay *Cassandra*, the nursing pioneer Florence Nightingale lambasted the Victorian family for the enforced idleness of its middle-class daughters. She led a team of nurses who served in Constantinople during the Crimean War (1854–1856), earning the moniker "The Lady with the Lamp," and her reforms involved designing new measures to help prevent infection (described in her 1859 book *Notes on Nursing: What It Is and What It Is Not*) as well as the establishment of the first professional school for nurses, the Nightingale Training School at St. Thomas Hospital, which opened its doors in 1860 (Poovey 1988).

In the 1850s and 1860s, societies like the Langham Place Circle and the Society for Promoting the Employment of Women began agitating for new forms of employment and education for middle-class women. However, a license to practice medicine remained largely the purview of men until the mid-1870s. Elizabeth Blackwell, born in Bristol, England and educated in America, became the first woman to receive a medical degree in the United States in 1849, and served as an inspiration to generations of aspiring female doctors in Britain (Blackwell 1895). Elizabeth Garrett Anderson qualified for a license in 1865 by passing the examination offered by the Society of Apothecaries, a loophole that was subsequently closed in an effort to discourage other women to follow in her footsteps. Undeterred, Garrett Anderson received a medical degree from the Sorbonne in Paris in 1870, all the while maintaining her own practice and the St. Mary's Dispensary for Women and Children (later renamed the New Hospital for Women), an institution specializing in offering medical and gynaecological care to poor women. With Sophia Jex-Blake, Garrett Anderson co-founded the London

School of Medicine for Women; Jex-Blake was another pioneering female physician, the first woman licensed to practice medicine in Scotland and a member of the "Edinburgh Seven," a group of women who matriculated at the University of Edinburgh in 1869 and campaigned for women's access to medical education (Crawford 2002). Women's struggles to advance their careers in medicine and nursing paralleled other feminist reform efforts of the period, and in many ways these campaigns symbolize a larger struggle against the normative ideologies of gender in the second half of the nineteenth century.

### *"Odd" Women: Heterosexuality, Normativity, and Difference*

The campaign for access to higher education and professional training for middle-class women occurred against the backdrop of debates over women's independence, employment, and marital status from the 1850s and 1860s through the 1890s. The 1851 census revealed a disparity of half a million more women than men, and such women were quickly labeled "superfluous" as a result of the likelihood that they would remain unmarried. Liberal manufacturer and industrialist W. R. Greg argued for female emigration and domestic service as a solution to the demographic problem posed by such so-called "odd" women; in fact, the more practicable solution was to reimagine the traditional approach to the education of girls and young women, and to reconceive the social stigma associated with spinsterhood (Martineau 1859; Greg 1862).

Much like the debate over "superfluous women" in the 1850s and 1860s, the phenomenon of the "New Woman" shaped late nineteenth-century discourses around gender norms (Figure 2.7). Originating in literary and visual media of the 1890s, this figure—an educated, mobile, empowered young woman who courted scandal by smoking cigarettes, riding bicycles, and most importantly, by challenging men's dominance in the public sphere—undermined earlier, more restrictive feminine ideals and opened up new possibilities for imagining different models of femininity and gender (Ardis 1990; Mitchell 1995; Garvey 1996; Nelson 2001; Richardson and Willis 2002). The New Woman became a cultural icon of increased social, sexual, economic and intellectual freedom, and her physical and social mobility in particular underscored the changing discourses around the body in the late Victorian era. Not only did such changes occur in the realm of women's dress—from undergarments like corsets and petticoats, to the length and shape of the skirt and the overall silhouette—as will be discussed further in subsequent chapters, but also in changing understandings of women's sexual subjectivity. The New Woman found a counterpart in the figure of the lesser-known "New Man," an enlightened male partner with feminist

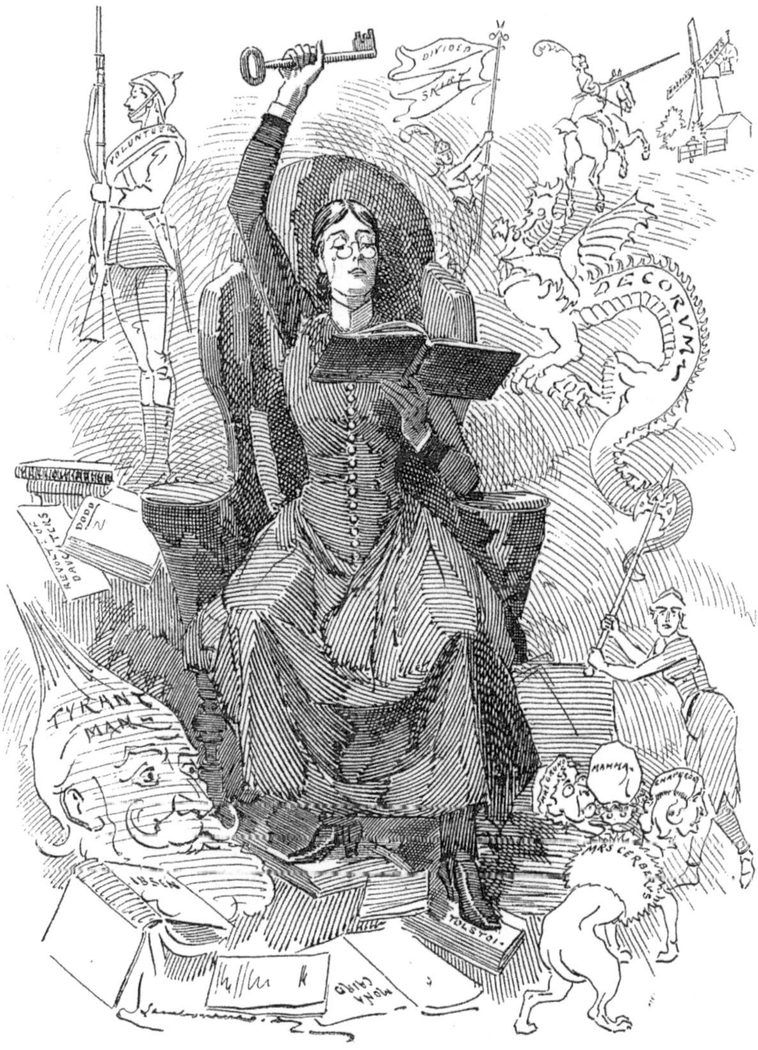


*Figure 2.7* “Donna Quixote.” *Punch,* 28 April 1894. Vol. 106, p. 194. Public domain. Courtesy of Williston Library, Mount Holyoke College.

leanings; she also embodied women’s ability to reject the dominant ideology of marriage as the endpoint of women’s lives.

As cultural norms around marriage and domesticity began to change, the figure of the spinster began to be reclaimed as an alternative to the dominant patriarchal and heteronormative ideology (Vicinus 1985; Liggins 2016). Likewise, although lesbianism was still subject to discrimination and stigmatization (if not legally, then culturally proscribed), women developed multiple approaches to female partnership throughout the era, from the "Boston marriages" of the later nineteenth century United States (Faderman 1981) to the "romantic friendships" and other forms of female partnership in Victorian Britain (Vicinus 2004; Marcus 2007). Recent research in the spheres of autobiography and life writing has uncovered a far wider range of Victorian sexual identities than the presumption of heterosexuality dictates. As letters and diaries reveal, not all those born female in the Victorian era identified as women, and not all those who identified as women were originally sexed female at birth. As research continues into the lives and experiences of lesbian, queer, transgender, and intersex people in the nineteenth century, we will be able to develop a much broader understanding of what it meant to experience life as a woman in Victorian Britain.

## To Sum Up

- Victorian scientists strove to use empirical (biological) data to create categories of human difference; but their interpretations were grounded in culturally bound assumptions about sexuality, gender, race, and class.
- Scientists constructed gender difference using their culturally laden interpretations of biological facts to develop the idea that the natural female body was inferior to the natural male body.
- The ideology of separate spheres laid out distinct realms for men and women; but Victorian moral codes meant that men and women were distinguished by sexual and moral differences.
- Victorian moral codes were bound up in legal and social realities that disenfranchised all women, some more than others.

## Questions to Consider

- How do the racially and gender-biased origins of Darwin's evolutionary theory call into question "objectivity" even as it is understood as a defining feature of modern science? Can we accept "objectivity" if these ideologies are still embedded in science, medicine, and culture today?
- If controlling sex workers' bodies resulted from scientific reasoning such as disease control, when did this desire for control shift to be more morally driven? Or was it always tied to the morality and purity that was considered a norm for Victorian women?
- How did religious ideas fuel and/or confirm how women were regarded in Victorian society?

## Notes

1 Although Darwin began developing these ideas as early as 1844, he refrained from publishing his work for over a decade, prompted to do so in part by research undertaken independently by the British naturalist Alfred Russel Wallace. Wallace's essay "On the Tendency of Varieties to Depart Indefinitely from the Original Type" was presented, alongside an unpublished piece by Darwin, to the Linnean Society of London in 1858.

2 Although Thomas Sydenham had identified hysterical symptoms in men, which he termed hypochondriasis, hysteria remained a primarily female-identified disease until the recognition that soldiers afflicted with shell shock during the First World War manifested similar symptoms: as Elaine Showalter notes, "the hysterical soldier was seen as simple, emotional, unthinking, passive, suggestible, dependent, and weak—very much the same constellation of traits associated with the hysterical woman" (Showalter 1985, 175).

## References

### *Primary Sources*

Beeton, Isabella. 1861. *The Book of Household Management*. London: S. O. Beeton.

Blackstone, William. 1765. *Commentaries on the Laws of England: In Four Books*. Adapted to the Present State of the Law by Robert Malcolm Kerr. Vol. I: Of the Rights of Persons. 3rd ed. London: John Murray, 1862.

Blackwell, Elizabeth. 1895. *Pioneer Work in Opening the Medical Profession to Women*. London/New York: Longmans, Green, and Co.

Brontë, Charlotte. 1847. *Jane Eyre*. Edited with an introduction by Richard Nemesvari. Peterborough, ON: Broadview Press, 1999.

Darwin, Charles. 1859. *On the Origin of Species*. London: John Murray.

Darwin, Charles. 1871. *The Descent of Man, and Selection in Relation to Sex*. London: John Murray.

Engelmann, George. 1882, 2nd ed. 1883. *Labor Among Primitive Peoples*. London: J. H. Chambers.

Galton, Francis. 1883. *Inquiries into Human Faculty and Its Development*. London: Macmillan and Co.

Geddes, Patrick, and J. Arthur Thompson. 1889. *The Evolution of Sex*. London: W. Scott.

Greg, W. R. 1862. "Why Are Women Redundant?" *National Review* (April). Reprinted in W. R. Greg, *Literary and Social Judgments*, 274–308. London: N. Trübner and Co, 1869.

Martineau, Harriet. 1859. "Female Industry." Reprinted in *Criminals, Idiots, Women, and Minors: Victorian Writing by Women on Women*, 29–73, edited by Susan Hamilton. Peterborough, ON: Broadview Press, 1995.

Mill, John Stuart. 1869. *The Subjection of Women*. In *The Basic Writings of John Stuart Mill*, 123–229. Edited with an introduction by J. B. Schneewind; notes and commentary by Dale E. Miller. New York: Modern Library, 2002.

Nightingale, Florence. 1852. *Cassandra.* Edited with an introduction by Myra Stark. New York: The Feminist Press, 1979.

Nightingale, Florence. 1859. *Notes on Nursing: What It Is, and What It Is Not.* With a foreword by Virginia M. Dunbar and a new preface by Margaret B. Dolan. Mineola, NY: Dover, 1969.

Smith, Barbara Leigh [later Bodichon]. 1854; 2nd ed. revised with additions, 1856. *A Brief Summary, in Plain Language, of the Most Important Laws Concerning Women; Together with a Few Observations Thereon.* London: John Chapman.

Wallace, Alfred Russel. 1858. "On the Tendency of Varieties to Depart Indefinitely from the Original Type." *Proceedings of the Linnaean Society of London* 3: 53–62.

### Secondary Sources

Anderson, Amanda. 1993. *Tainted Souls and Painted Faces: The Rhetoric of Fallenness in Victorian Culture.* 2018 rev. ed. Ithaca, NY: Cornell University Press.

Ardis, Ann. 1990. "Preliminaries: Naming the New Woman." In Ann Ardis, *New Women, New Novels: Feminism and Early Modernism*, 10–28. New Brunswick, NJ: Rutgers University Press.

Briggs, Laura. 2000. "The Race of Hysteria: 'Overcivilization' and the 'Savage' Woman in Late Nineteenth-Century Obstetrics and Gynecology." *American Quarterly* 52 (2): 246–273.

Cannon-Mohammed, Zara. 2018. "Examining Difference: The Neuroscience of Sex and the History of Gender Roles." Unpublished Division III Thesis. Amherst, MA: Hampshire College.

Copelman, Dina M. 1996. *London's Women Teachers: Gender, Class, and Feminism, 1870–1930.* New York: Routledge.

Crais, Clifton, and Pamela Scully. *Sara Baartman and the Hottentot Venus: A Ghost Story and a Biography.* Princeton: Princeton University Press, 2009.

Crawford, Elizabeth. 2002. *Enterprising Women: The Garretts and Their Circle.* London: Francis Boutle.

Dames, Nicholas. 2001. "Amnesiac Bodies: Phrenology, Physiology, and Memory in Charlotte Brontë." In Nicholas Dames, *Amnesiac Selves: Nostalgia, Forgetting, and British Fiction, 1810–1870*, 76–124. Oxford: Oxford University Press.

Davidoff, Leonore, and Catherine Hall. 1987. *Family Fortunes: Men and Women of the English Middle Class 1780–1850.* 2002 rev. ed. London: Hutchinson. Abingdon: Routledge.

Davin, Anna. 1978. "Imperialism and Motherhood." *History Workshop Journal* 5 (1): 9–66.

Elliott, Paul. 2003. "Erasmus Darwin, Herbert Spencer, and the Origins of the Evolutionary Worldview in British Provincial Scientific Culture, 1770–1850." *Isis* 94 (1): 1–29.

Faderman, Lillian. 1981. *Surpassing the Love of Men.* London: The Women's Press.

Fischer-Tiné, Harald, and Michael Mann, eds. 2004. *Colonialism as Civilizing Mission: Cultural Ideology in British India.* London: Anthem Press.

Garvey, Ellen Gruber. 1996. "Reframing the Bicycle: Magazines and Scorching Women." In Ellen Gruber Garvey, *The Adman in the Parlor: Magazines and the Gendering of Consumer Culture*, 106–134. Oxford: Oxford University Press.

Gilman, Sander L. 1985. "Black Bodies, White Bodies: Toward an Iconography of Female Sexuality in Late Nineteenth-Century Art, Medicine, and Literature." *Critical Inquiry* 12 (1): 204–242.

Hallam, Julia. 2000. *Nursing the Image: Media, Culture, and Professional Identity*. London/New York: Routledge.

Harvey, Karen. 2002. "The Century of Sex? Gender, Bodies, and Sexuality in the Long Eighteenth Century." *The Historical Journal* 45 (4): 899–916.

Hawkins, Sue. 2010. *Nursing and Women's Labour in the Nineteenth Century: The Quest for Independence*. London/New York: Routledge.

Helsinger, Elizabeth K., Robin Lauterbach Sheets, and William Veeder, eds. 1983. *The Woman Question: Society and Literature in Britain and America, 1837–1883*. 3 vols. New York: Garland Publishing.

Homans, Margaret, and Adrienne Munich, eds. 1997. *Remaking Queen Victoria*. Cambridge: Cambridge University Press.

Jordan, Jane. 2007. *Josephine Butler*. London: Hambledon Continuum.

Judd, Catherine. 1998. *Bedside Seductions: Nursing and the Victorian Imagination, 1830–1880*. New York: St. Martin's Press.

Langland, Elizabeth. 1995. *Nobody's Angels: Middle-Class Women and Domestic Ideology in Victorian Culture*. Ithaca, NY: Cornell University Press, 1995.

Laqueur, Thomas W. 1990. *Making Sex: Body and Gender from the Greeks to Freud*. Cambridge, MA: Harvard University Press.

Liggins, Emma. 2016. *Odd Women? Spinsters, Lesbians and Widows in British Women's Fiction, 1850s–1930s*. Manchester: Manchester University Press.

Lewontin, Richard C. 1983. "Biological Determinism." *Tanner Lectures on Human Values* 4: 147–183.

Logan, Deborah. 2010. *Harriet Martineau, Victorian Imperialism, and the Civilizing Mission*. Farnham: Ashgate.

Marcus, Sharon. 2007. *Between Women: Friendship, Desire, and Marriage in Victorian England*. Princeton, NJ: Princeton University Press.

Micale, Mark S. 1995. *Approaching Hysteria: Disease and Its Interpretations*. Princeton, NJ: Princeton University Press.

Mitchell, Sally. 1995. *The New Girl: Girls' Culture in England, 1880–1915*. New York: Columbia University Press.

Munich, Adrienne. 1996. *Queen Victoria's Secrets*. New York: Columbia University Press.

Nelson, Carolyn Christensen, ed. 2001. *A New Woman Reader: Fiction, Articles, and Drama of the 1890s*. Peterborough, ON: Broadview Press.

Netto, Priscilla. 2005. "Reclaiming the Body of the 'Hottentot': The Vision and Visuality of the Body Speaking with Vengeance in Venus Hottentot 2000." *European Journal of Women's Studies* 12 (2): 149–163.

Petrie, Glen. 1971. *A Singular Iniquity: The Campaigns of Josephine Butler*. London: Macmillan.

Poovey, Mary. 1988. *Uneven Developments: The Ideological Work of Gender in Mid-Victorian England.* Chicago, IL: University of Chicago Press.

Richardson, Angelique, and Chris Wills, eds. 2001. *The New Woman in Fiction and in Fact: Fin-de-Siècle Feminisms*. Houndsmills, Basingstoke, Hampshire: Palgrave Macmillan.

Rubinstein, David. 1991. *A Different World for Women: The Life of Millicent Garrett Fawcett*. Columbus, OH: Ohio State University Press.

Said, Edward. 1993. *Culture and Imperialism*. New York: Knopf.

Sanders, Lise Shapiro. 2015. "'Equal Laws Based Upon an Equal Standard': The Garrett Sisters, the Contagious Diseases Acts, and the Sexual Politics of Victorian and Edwardian Feminism Revisited." *Women's History Review* 24 (3): 389–409.

Schiebinger, Londa. 1986. "Skeletons in the Closet: The First Illustrations of the Female Skeleton in Eighteenth-Century Anatomy." *Representations* (14): 42–82.

Schiebinger, Londa. 1993. "Why Mammals Are Called Mammals: Gender Politics in Eighteenth-Century Natural History." *The American Historical Review* 98 (2): 382–411.

Showalter, Elaine. 1985. *The Female Malady: Women, Madness, and English Culture, 1830–1980*. New York: Penguin.

Steinbach, Susie L. 2012; 2nd ed. 2017. *Understanding the Victorians: Politics, Culture and Society in Nineteenth-Century Britain.* London/New York: Routledge.

Stepan, Nancy. 1982. *The Idea of Race in Science: Great Britain, 1800–1960.* Houndsmills, Basingstoke, Hampshire: Macmillan.

Vicinus, Martha. 1985. *Independent Women: Work and Community for Single Women 1850–1920*. Chicago, IL: University of Chicago Press.

Vicinus, Martha. 2004. *Intimate Friends: Women Who Loved Women, 1778–1928.* Chicago, IL: University of Chicago Press.

Walkowitz, Judith. 1980. *Prostitution and Victorian Society: Women, Class, and the State*. Cambridge: Cambridge University Press.

Walsh, Anthony, and Ellis, Lee. 2006. *Criminology: An Interdisciplinary Approach.* London: Sage.

Welter, Barbara. 1976. "The Cult of True Womanhood." In Barbara Welter, *Dimity Convictions: The American Woman in the Nineteenth Century*, 21–41. Athens, OH: Ohio University Press.

## *Online Sources*

The National Archives."Research Guide to Asylums, Psychiatric Hospitals, and Mental Health." Available at: http://www.nationalarchives.gov.uk/help-with-your-research/research-guides/mental-health/. Accessed 20 September 2019.

White, Tim. 2019. "Evolution of Evolution: Human Evolution's Winding Path." National Science Foundation Flash Special Report: https://www.nsf.gov/news/special_reports/darwin/textonly/anthro_essay2.jsp. Accessed 7 August 2019.

# 3 Girlhood, Adolescence, and Sexuality

## Introduction

In this chapter we address the biocultural contexts of health and wellness for girls and young women in the Victorian period. Beginning with a discussion of discourses around education, we analyze the heated debate over whether women's bodies—their anatomy and physiology, particularly with respect to reproduction—affected their ability to receive an education equal to that of their male peers. We then delve more deeply into the lives of working-class girls and women in the nineteenth century, exploring the impact of factory work and the legislative changes that affected female health and wellness. From a biocultural perspective we consider both direct and indirect measures of health and wellness in industrial England, paying particular attention to the epidemic of rickets and its impact, and what such measures can reveal about the lived experience of being female in the Victorian era. Studying health and disease in the nineteenth century, and the social and environmental conditions that put women of all classes at risk for increased morbidity and mortality, offers a useful set of insights into cultural discourses around the female body. By analyzing the widespread use of corsets and other measures to obtain the ideal silhouette dictated by the fashions of the era, we gain insight into how women were controlled and considered within the social fabric of Victorian society. In conclusion, we investigate later nineteenth-century efforts to reform fashion by altering the restrictive garments worn by most women, examining how such social reforms led to greater social mobility for girls and young women. Our analysis in this chapter paves the way for a discussion in Chapter 4 of marriage, motherhood, and health for women during the childbearing years.

## Education and the Debate Over Women's Minds and Bodies

As noted in Chapters 1 and 2, Victorian science was structured through an understanding of human variation, evolution, and theories of civilization and racial progress that took the white male body as the norm against which all other bodies were defined. As a result, white female bodies were placed at the center of a set of discourses that framed their importance to narratives of reproduction, particularly the reproduction of citizens of the British imperial nation (Davin 1978). Victorian medical texts, popular literature, periodicals, and even advertising conveyed an extremely limited feminine ideal based on notions of whiteness, fragility, and delicacy that had significant effects on both the lives and the bodies of Victorian girls and young women. Beginning at an early age, girls and young women were taught to take up their proper role within the family, as caretakers and guardians of morality (Dyhouse 1981; McDermid 2012). They were also encouraged to see themselves as little wives and mothers in the making, and to that end, they were exhorted to protect their bodies, and especially their reproductive systems, from harm. In this section, we outline Victorian perspectives on education as they affected girls and young women, and explore the debate in the 1870s over higher education for women, which turned on Victorian conceptions of the fragile white female body that were in turn shaped by theories of racial hierarchy outlined in previous chapters.

### *Educating the Victorian Girl*

For much of the Victorian period, education took place in the home. In working- and middle-class homes, mothers would teach young children the fundamentals of reading, writing, and arithmetic; in upper-class homes, such tasks would fall to domestic caretakers (nannies and nursemaids). While many children did attend local grammar, charity, or "dame" schools (so called after their headmistresses), formal schooling was dependent on availability and familial resources. It was not until the 1870 Education Act that school boards were formalized to provide and supervise teaching in non-denominational "board schools," and another decade passed before such schooling was made compulsory in the 1880 Education Act. Fees were required until 1891, and subsequent legislation elevated the minimum required school-leaving age to 11 (in 1893) and 12 (in 1899).

Children from wealthy families were privately educated, with a governess or tutor taking responsibility for the elementary education of both boys and girls. In early adolescence, male children of the titled and landowning classes would attend a "public" or independent school (paradoxically, a private form of schooling based on tuition and independent of state and local schools), while female children were typically educated at home throughout their teenage years (Fletcher 2008). Alternatively, young women might be sent to academies emphasizing the skills and talents needed to succeed as wives, mothers, and guardians of the domestic sphere. In her 1839 treatise *The Women of England, Their Social Duties and Domestic Habits*, Sarah Stickney Ellis argued for the importance of an education that would serve as the foundation for a young woman's character, befitting women's role as caretakers (Ellis 1839). Women were expected to demonstrate a superficial knowledge of history, geography, and languages, and to develop their talents in music, drawing and other fine arts, and needlework; yet these were considered by many merely as mechanisms through which to increase a young woman's attractiveness to male suitors rather than developing their character and intellect. Elizabeth Barrett Browning's 1857 verse novel *Aurora Leigh* wryly characterizes the limitations of such an education, given to the protagonist by her aunt: "I learnt a little algebra, a little/Of the mathematics,—brushed with extreme flounce/The circle of the sciences [...] Spun glass, stuffed birds, and modelled flowers in wax/Because she liked accomplishments in girls" (Barrett Browning 1857, Book I, ll. 403–405, 425–426). An education of this kind enabled young women to participate in society, but did not equip them for independent employment. The fact that many middle-class women who sought to earn their own living had few options other than teaching speaks to the reality that during the early to mid-Victorian period, most women were not educated for a life beyond marriage and child-rearing.

## *Sex, Gender, and Higher Education*

Educational reformers, among them the feminist pioneers who founded the first women's colleges in Britain in the late 1860s and 1870s, were strongly critical of the narrow education most Victorian girls and young women received. Emily Davies, co-founder of Girton College, Cambridge, legal scholar Barbara Leigh Smith Bodichon, Dr. Elizabeth Garrett (later Anderson), and many others strove to combat the mid-Victorian view of women's unsuitability for higher education and professional careers (Davies 1866; Caine 1992; Gordon and Doughan 2001; Lacey 2001). In so doing, they supported the nascent feminist movement, and laid the groundwork for the suffrage campaign throughout the remaining decades of the nineteenth century (Jordan 1999; Sanders 2015).

The debate over women's education engaged questions of women's mental and physical health, with particular attention to their preparedness for the challenges of higher education. This debate intensified with the publication of Edward Hammond Clarke's *Sex in Education: A Fair Chance for the Girls* (1873). Dr. Clarke, a professor at Harvard University's medical school from 1855 to 1872, originally presented his argument as a lecture to the New England Woman's Club in Boston, Massachusetts, exhorting audience members to exercise caution in pursuing their education lest they suffer from the "evil effects of continuous mental work on women's health" (Clarke 1873). In reply, Louise S. Hotchkiss, a Boston teacher and author of essays on women and education, wrote an article called "Corsets, Versus Brains," published in the *Cambridge Chronicle* on 8 March 1873. In this piece, Hotchkiss critiqued the position of "learned male physicians" concerning the physical and mental condition of women, and pointed to numerous examples of "strong, healthy-minded, and healthy-bodied women" who withstood the challenges of mental labor with no ill effects. Instead, Hotchkiss blamed corsetry and women's restrictive clothing for the debilitating burden placed on the female body, and argues for a "reform in dress" to free women from such constraints (a topic to be further explored in the next section).

In an 1874 article for the *Fortnightly Review* entitled "Sex in Mind and in Education," the British psychiatrist Henry Maudsley, influenced by Edward Clarke's book, presented a similar argument that the physiological differences between the sexes rendered women unfit for the rigors of mental labor associated with university education. In his view, the "tyranny" of women's physiology following the onset of puberty marked out a specific terrain of physical and mental differences that structured women's separate identity and sphere of influence, leading him to conclude that "there is sex in mind as well as sex in body" (Maudsley 1874, 466). Maudsley argued for an "adapted" education for women, specifically designed to attend "to the peculiarities of their constitution, to the special functions in life for which they are destined, and to the range and kind of practical activity, mental and bodily, to which they would seem to be foreordained by their sexual organization of body and mind" (1874, 483).

Dr. Elizabeth Garrett Anderson, herself married and a mother as well as a licensed physician in 1874, published a reply to Maudsley articulating the value of women's higher education. Garrett Anderson argued that, rather than suffering from the rigors of higher education, women benefited from the intellectual stimulation and companionship that offered a welcome alternative to the "dullness" provoked by a lack of meaningful work. For Garrett Anderson, the new system of women's education, which incorporated a common goal but enabled men and women to attain it "each in their own way, and without the stimulus of daily rivalry" (1874, 593), offered numerous benefits for women's mental and physical constitution. Garrett Anderson tactically used Maudsley's taxonomy of sexual difference to establish new ways of conceiving of women's physiology and capacity for mental labor. Her reply appears on the surface to embrace existing categories of gender and sexual difference, but suggests a deeper, seismic shift in Victorian conceptions of women's intellectual and professional abilities.

As the above examples suggest, Victorian doctors worked in an environment that encouraged them to think of physiology, behavior, character traits, and even cognitive ability as biologically structured through differences of sex. Our next section addresses the ways in which physiology was affected by differences of class in the Victorian era, especially in the context of industrialization; and we pay particular attention to the ways in which discourses around health and wellness affected the bodies and lives of Victorian girls and young women.

## Class and Health

### *Labor and Legislation*

Victorian work encompassed a variety of occupations—from agricultural and industrial labor (farms, mines, mills), to factory and shop work, to office work, to the professions, as well domestic service (the latter was a major employer of young people as well as adults). Much of Victorian labor was categorized by the relationship of the worker to systems of production and distribution, and the nineteenth century as a whole was characterized by the development of industrial capitalism and the struggle for equitable treatment for workers. Various pieces of legislation, including the 1834 Poor Law Amendment Act and several Factory Acts passed throughout the remainder of the century, had a dramatic impact on improvements in public health, although Victorian women and children (and men) of the working classes still struggled with the negative effects of long hours, insufficient nutrition, low pay, and overwork. Meanwhile, the middle and upper classes espoused an ideology of uplift that maintained the existing class structure while extending the reach of philanthropy and social reform into the lives of working people.

The effects of urbanization and the growth of industrial capitalism resulted in an ever-growing disparity between the rich and the poor, which is reflected in studies of health and disease during this period. Key pieces of legislation passed in the early 1830s included the New Poor Law of 1834, which resulted in the creation of workhouses under the supervision of local boards of governors. The intentionally harsh conditions in the Victorian workhouse were designed to motivate people to seek alternatives in the form of regular paid employment. However, the conditions in workhouses and the social stigma associated with them, not to mention the real economic disparities of industrial capitalism, resulted in widespread concern over the issue of poverty and its effects on public health and disease.

We can grasp the effects of the harsh realities of the workhouse on the bodies of the poor through direct studies of urban populations at this time. Scholarship examining stature (height) from those living (Harris 1998, 2008), mortality statistics which were in their infancy (Dobbie 1982; Loudon 1997), as well as stature and pathological skeletal analyses when cemeteries are moved (Mays et al. 2008; Nitsch et al. 2011; DeWitte et al. 2016) has been considered against the backdrop of an economic analysis to assess how the disparities between the rich and poor impacted both lived experience and life expectancy. The case can be made that throughout the Victorian period, social inequalities, as evidenced through these different entry points, can be seen in the increases in rates of infant mortality, shorter heights, poorer health, and lower life expectancies for the poor (Newman and Gowland 2017). In addition, the 1840s and 1850s marked an era of unparalleled social analysis as new approaches to policy and public health led to numerous investigations and exposés of the poverty and ill health of a wide swath of the population (Chadwick 1842; Engels 1845; Mayhew 1851). The "Condition of England" novelists of the 1840s—among them Charles Dickens, Benjamin Disraeli, and Elizabeth Gaskell—used fictional narratives as an opportunity to expose the dangers of urbanization and the exploitation of workers, and contributed to the success of reform efforts in subsequent decades.

Girls and young women were dramatically affected by the conditions of daily life for poor and working-class people in Victorian England. Although childhood as a concept was still evolving throughout this period (Nelson 1999), children were considered workers from a very early age, whether in caring for siblings and tending to the home, or in working outside the home as agricultural and industrial laborers (and within it as domestic servants) (Steinbach 2004). Domestic service remained an unregulated trade throughout the century, and girls as young as ten would be recruited from workhouses or drawn from the families of tenants on landed estates to serve as scullery maids, maids-of-all-work, or in the nursery caring for their employers' children (Higgs 1983). Long hours and overwork were common in such environments, where one's tenure was also at the whim of the employer. Factory labor was similarly difficult, with employers enabled to pay lower wages to child workers who also risked physical endangerment due to exhaustion from ten- and twelve-hour workdays, exacerbated by nutritional insufficiency, ill health, and poor working conditions.

Skeletal and medical analyses have revealed a great deal about the complex health issues that poor children faced as they worked to survive (Lewis 2002; Newman and Gowland 2016). Many of the materials used in nineteenth-century factories were hazardous to the health of workers, among them the mercury used in making men's felt hats and in the quicksilvering of mirrors; lead, which was present in cosmetics as well as in paint; and arsenic, known to be poisonous but nonetheless present in everything from curtains and wallpaper to the green dyes used in artificial flowers and wreaths, dresses, and gloves (Teleky 1948; Malone 2003; Whorton 2010; Mathews David 2015). The *British Medical Journal* lamented, "A lady in full dress, duly decorated with a modern wreath of fifty green leaves, carries on her head forty grains of white arsenic—enough to poison herself and nineteen friends" (15 February 1862) (Figure 3.1).

These fashionable articles of clothing were undoubtedly dangerous to the women who wore them, but even more dangerous to the young women who made them. The artificial flower industry, and the dressmaking trades more generally, employed significant numbers of young women, who were nominally considered an asset for their dexterity with fine needlework while also seen as a cheaper form of labor (Jowitt and McIvor 1988; Greenlees 2007). As scientific understandings of environmental toxins and industrial pollutants progressed, activists began to advocate for the regulation of trades involving hazardous materials, and by the end of the century a

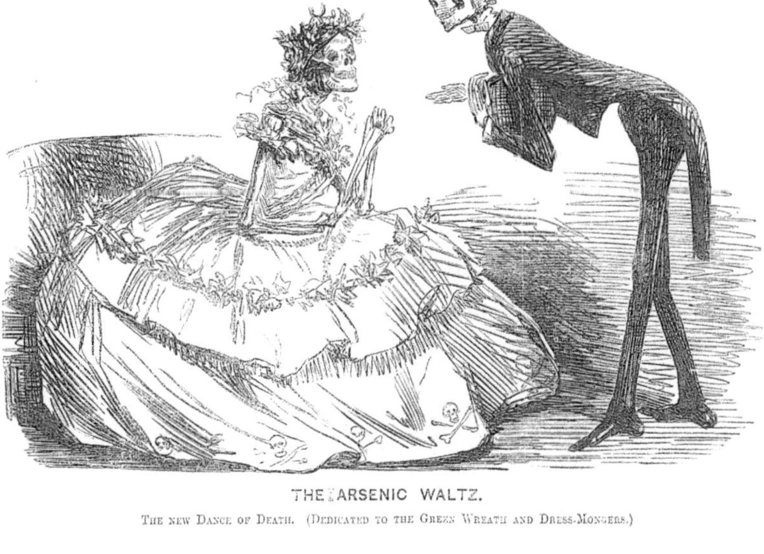

THE ARSENIC WALTZ.
THE NEW DANCE OF DEATH. (DEDICATED TO THE GREEN WREATH AND DRESS-MONGERS.)

*Figure 3.1* "The Arsenic Waltz." *Punch*, 8 February 1862. Vol. 42, p. 54. Courtesy of Williston Library, Mount Holyoke College.

commission was formed to regulate "dangerous trades" and bring health protections to workers (Oliver 1902; Harrison 1996; Nash 2015).

Prior to the Victorian era, school-age children were allowed to work in the textile mills and factories in the industrial North. The 1833 Factory Act prohibited the textile industry from employing children under the age of nine, limiting the length of the workday to eight hours for young people aged 9 to 13, and 12 hours for those 13 to 18 years of age (1833 Factory Act). Children under the age of 13 were also required to receive two hours of schooling per day. Factories were asked to comply with age certification requirements, and a team of factory inspectors enforced the new legislation. Inspectors' reports of abuses led to additional legislation in subsequent decades: modifications in 1844 further limited employment for children ages 8 to 13 and abolished the practice of employing women and children to work night shifts, and in 1847 women and children under the age of 18 were limited to ten-hour workdays (Nardinelli 1980).

In the 1860s, additional industries were brought under the purview of existing legislation; by 1867 any organization employing more than 50 people had to abide by the regulations of the Factory Acts. The Education Acts of 1870 and 1876 (described in further detail below) also affected the lives of young female workers, as education was mandated for children up to the age of ten, and the Factory Acts of 1891 and 1901 limited the minimum age of employment to 11, and then 12. In summary, extensive legislative efforts over the course of decades served to regulate the exploitation of young people in a range of industries, but the lengthy work day, combined with low wages and lack of nutritious food and exercise, prompted continuing concerns around the health and well-being of young people, which in turn led to various forms of protective legislation, including parliamentary committees on particular industries, as well as broader efforts to engage female workers in the emerging labor movement.

### *A Biocultural Case Study: London's Matchgirls*

Evidence of the adverse effects of developing industrial technologies on girls' and women's health can be seen through the success of the matchstick industry, which saw an upswing in the Victorian period with a new technology, white phosphorous, that allowed for a "strike-anywhere" match. We know today that the factories that were producing this high-demand product, such as the Bryant & May factory in East London, were primarily staffed with girls and young women (Satre 1982) (Figure 3.2).

These women and children suffered the multiple and long-term effects of toxic phosphorous inhalation, which included: cough, sputum production, and hemoptysis ("phossy lung"), systemic toxicity developed in the

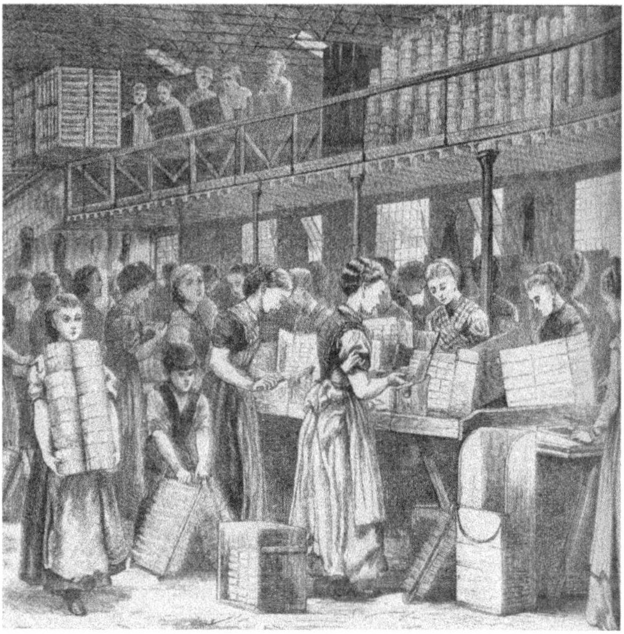

*Figure 3.2* Women working in a match factory in London in 1871. Public domain.

more chronically afflicted, provoking seizures ("phossy brain") and causing leukopenia and anemia ("phossy marrow"), and the phosphorous necrosis of the jaw where the bones of the jaw literally rot away ("phossy jaw") (see Figures 3.3 and 3.4) (Roberts et al. 2016; Gowland 2018; Gowland et al. 2018; Pollock et al. 2015). The dangers of working in this trade, combined with the long hours, low pay, and an exploitative system of fining workers for rule violations, led ultimately to a series of workers' actions in the 1870s and 1880s, including a petition presented to Parliament and a series of strikes.

The 1888 strike at the Bryant & May factory, popularly known as the matchgirls' strike, finally resulted in the abolition of the fine system and the provision of a separate room for meals that would help workers avoid contamination (Raw 2011). The Salvation Army opened its own factory in 1891, advertising its operation on "anti-sweating" (fair labor) and "health preserving" principles, although it struggled to succeed given the higher cost of its red phosphorous matches. As a result of the competition and negative publicity, Bryant & May eventually ceased using white phosphorous in 1901, and the House of Commons ultimately outlawed the use of

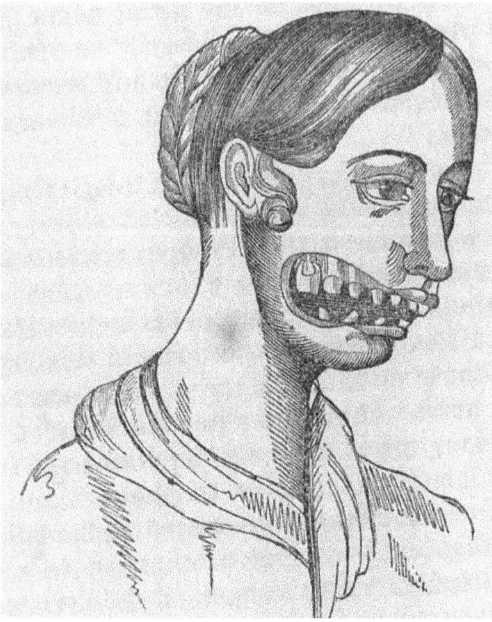

*Figure 3.3* 1896 drawing of phossy jaw by Mutter. Credit: Wikimedia Commons, CC BY-SA 4.0: https://commons.wikimedia.org/wiki/File:Phossy_jaw.jpg

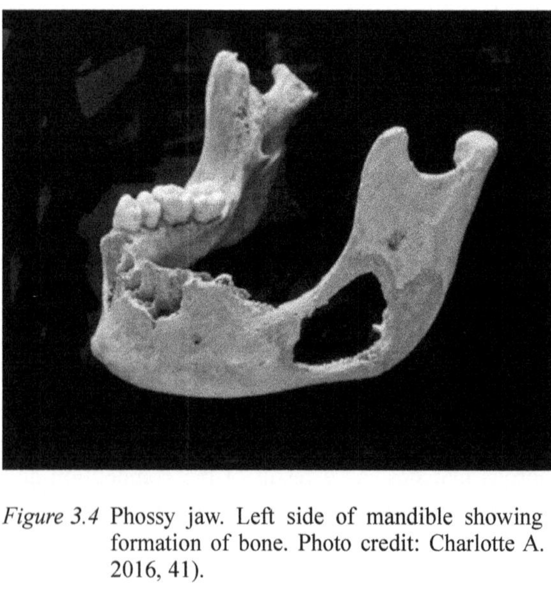

*Figure 3.4* Phossy jaw. Left side of mandible showing lateral destruction and formation of bone. Photo credit: Charlotte A. Roberts (Roberts et al. 2016, 41).

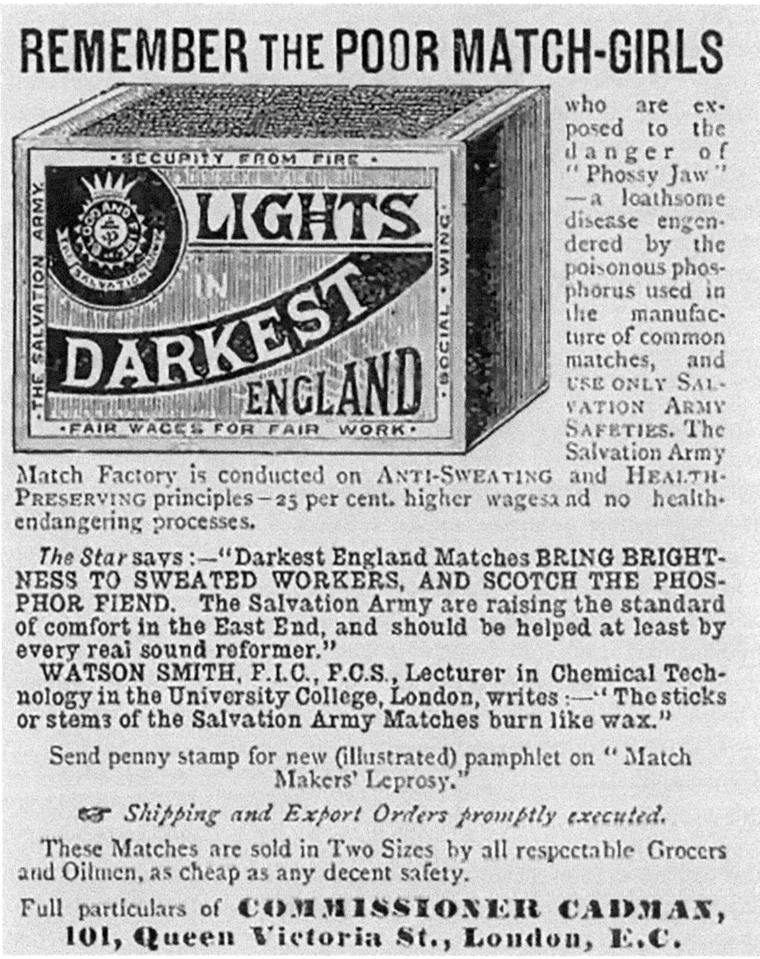
REMEMBER THE POOR MATCH-GIRLS
who are exposed to the danger of "Phossy Jaw"—a loathsome disease engendered by the poisonous phosphorus used in the manufacture of common matches, and USE ONLY SALVATION ARMY SAFETIES. The Salvation Army Match Factory is conducted on ANTI-SWEATING and HEALTH-PRESERVING principles—25 per cent. higher wages and no health-endangering processes.
SECURITY FROM FIRE
LIGHTS IN DARKEST ENGLAND
THE SALVATION ARMY
SOCIAL WING
FAIR WAGES FOR FAIR WORK
*The Star* says:—"Darkest England Matches BRING BRIGHTNESS TO SWEATED WORKERS, AND SCOTCH THE PHOSPHOR FIEND. The Salvation Army are raising the standard of comfort in the East End, and should be helped at least by every real sound reformer."
WATSON SMITH, F.I.C., F.C.S., Lecturer in Chemical Technology in the University College, London, writes:—"The sticks or stems of the Salvation Army Matches burn like wax."
Send penny stamp for new (illustrated) pamphlet on "Match Makers' Leprosy."
*Shipping and Export Orders promptly executed.*
These Matches are sold in Two Sizes by all respectable Grocers and Oilmen, as cheap as any decent safety.
Full particulars of COMMISSIONER CADMAN, 101, Queen Victoria St., London, E.C.

*Figure 3.5* Advertisement for Salvation Army safety matches, c. 1890s. Public domain.

white phosphorous in 1910, in keeping with the terms of the 1906 Berne Convention (Emsley 2004) (Figure 3.5).

In addition to the role played by efforts to improve the health and safety of girls and young women employed in factories, Victorian debates over factory and industrial labor engaged questions of girls' and young women's general state of health and preparedness to be in the workplace. The various pieces of legislation described above operated according to an ideological double standard that maintained class and gender norms. Middle-class white women, and their counterparts in the landed gentry and aristocracy, were considered members of the "weaker sex", more vulnerable to physical debility and disease than men of their social milieu. They were also seen to be more at risk for diseases such as hysteria and neurasthenia, which were culturally understood as feminine conditions, with some exceptions for the overtaxed existence of urban "brain workers" and, later, World War I veterans subject to shell shock (Mitchell 1871; Showalter 1985). Yet working-class women were not subject to such gendered assumptions, and were masculinized in the media as a result. Nonetheless, working-class women and children were vulnerable to the effects of malnutrition, exhaustion, and overwork that were particular to life in urban industrial areas (Levine-Clark 2004).

### *Measuring Health and Wellness in the Industrial World*

Current research into Victorian anatomy and physiology, especially the evidence that can be gleaned from studying the bones, can tell us much about health and wellness during the era of industrialization. Direct forms of study include a number of anthropometric measurements that can be taken on living individuals or on skeletal remains. Of particular interest is the role of height (stature), which has been shown to reveal key insights into the wellness of a community. Acute and long-term nutritional stresses during childhood can result in a decrease in stature, which in turn can be correlated to social and environmental factors: as Steckel argues, "Differences in height are related to improvements in diet, reductions in physical workloads, and to better health care" (Steckel 1995, 1991). For an understanding of Victorian female bodies and lives, evaluating stature presents a series of complications: prescribed by social codes, wealthier women were expected to eat less and to refrain from participating in any physical labor, while poor women were expected to work hard despite limited access to food. Thus, we would expect to see smaller stature for women in all classes during the Victorian period, resulting from decreased nutritional intake across the board. However, finding clear evidence of differences in stature for Victorian women is difficult, as most studies were conducted on soldiers, or on institutionalized individuals (criminals and asylum patients, for example). These demographics only offer a glimpse of the actual stature for people of the time; one can infer that they may not reflect the general public, and cannot be clearly tied to class; moreover, most often they reflect male rather than female health.

#### *Stature*

Stature (height) is a direct measure that can be used to assess the relationship between socioeconomics and nutritional access. It is well documented that at key periods in growth and development, chronic malnutrition and/or infections can impede individuals from reaching their full height potential (Cameron and Demerath 2002; Dansforth et al. 2011). As Dansforth et al. (2011) note, "[a]dult height is considered to represent the cumulative effects of growth and development and regularly serves as a proxy of general, non-specific population health, both in the present and in the skeletal remains of past populations" (377). A number of stature studies done on English soldiers (or the boys being recruited) that directly measured living heights or that were completed through skeletal analysis show that there was a decline in height as the industrialization of England took place beginning in the eighteenth century and continuing into the Victorian era (Horrell et al. 1998; Komlos, 1993, 1998) (Figure 3.6).

These studies consider socioeconomics, household make-up, and nutritional access on the overall stature of boys and men. But they do not consider the social frameworks that are often at work, in which boys are offered more food over their sisters, and mothers often go without to feed their children and maintain households (Horrell et al. 1998).

Studies that focus on direct measurements of female stature during industrialization are limited, as females (and more specifically elite white females) were not often included in large-scale studies, and when they were, they were often criminals who were incarcerated or in asylums (Komlos 1998). In addition, there is a paucity of studies that offer direct

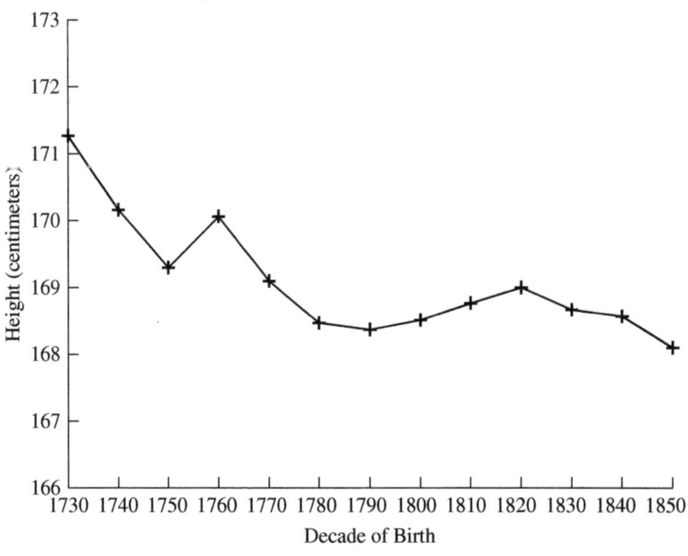


*Figure 3.6* "Height of English soldiers, 20–23 years old" (Komlos 1998, 781).

skeletal measurements for female stature from archaeological sources. Thus to begin to understand the impact of industrialization directly on female stature requires other tools of analysis. For the poor we can infer that female height followed the same decreases as their male counterparts of the times (and may have been more dramatic as poor females had a larger burden of nutritional deficiencies); but with the lack of direct anthropometric analysis we need to devise other ways to consider health impacts on poor women.

We know that nutritional deficiencies, combined with cultural behaviors and environmental issues resulting from industrialization, had marked effects on the Victorian female body, including on stature. In addition, the shift from an agricultural to an industrial economy, changing patterns of daily living, including changes to working and housing conditions, meant that working people had less exposure to sunlight as a result of working indoors (in factories, shops, and homes) and living in crowded urban tenements. The increasingly powerful ideology of domesticity likewise resulted in a decrease of time spent outdoors for middle-class white women, who were also encouraged to protect their skin from the sun. The lack of sun exposure, combined with poor nutrition, resulted in an epidemic of extremely high rates of metabolic diseases such as rickets.

### *Rickets*

Rickets is a disorder resulting from severe vitamin D deficiency that primarily affects children (Mayo Clinic 2019). When extreme and prolonged, rickets impacts proper bone development. When nutrition is compromised at an early age and is long-term and chronic, susceptibility to rickets is increased, resulting in what is called long-bone bowing. Such alterations of the bone structure have profound effects on skeletal shape and size, reverberating into adulthood.

Rickets occurs when there is inadequate nutrition or sun exposure, as vitamin D is most effectively synthesized through the skin as a result of exposure to the UV rays of the sun (Lips 2006). Vitamin D is essential to the proper mineralization of bone during growth and development (Theobald 2005; Brickley and Ives 2008; Wells et al. 2012), and in adults severe deficiency causes osteomalacia, where the new bone, the osteoid, is not mineralized (Lips 2006). Research today also links adequate vitamin D to the prevention of autoimmune diseases and some cancers (Lips 2006).

Chronic childhood rickets can impact critical growth and development and has a lasting effect on the shape of the legs and pelvic girdle, which impact overall stature (Brickley and Ives 2008; Wells et al. 2012). The condition of "rachitis" (as rickets was termed in the nineteenth century) has been documented over the centuries and across the globe. During the Victorian period in Great Britain, children in particular experienced extremely high rates of rickets, perhaps the worst epidemic of rickets ever documented (Gibbs 1994; Hardy 1992; Loudon 1992).

Figure 3.7 shows how Victorian children with extreme, chronic rachitis bones would look. Here we can see how the long bones softened by rickets take on an inward or outward bow-shape. This distortion of the long bones is not only visible in childhood, but when the cases are extreme, even when

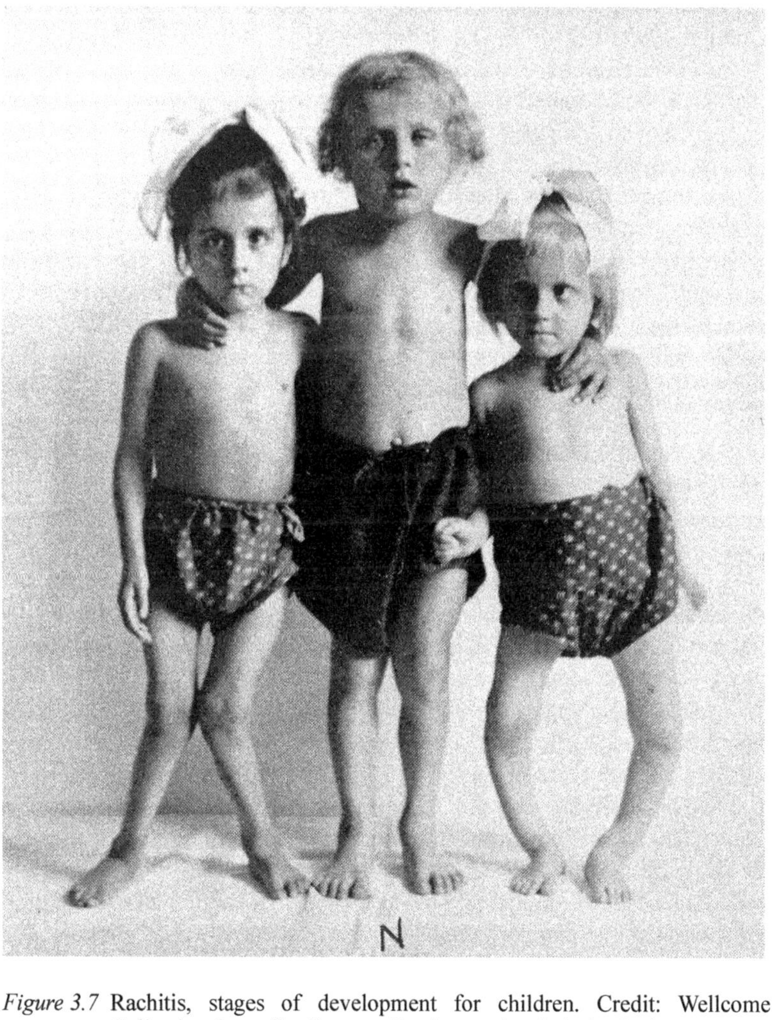


*Figure 3.7* Rachitis, stages of development for children. Credit: Wellcome Collection. https://wellcomecollection.org/works/m3eu5snb

the deficiency is managed, the overall shape changes of the bones will not resolve and the adult will have a bow of the legs. The result of this is that as a child with chronic rickets grows, stature will be compromised for life.

Rickets can also impact the bones of the pelvis. The deformities caused by rachitis have been categorized as a "rickety flat pelvis," in which the bones of the pelvic girdle (innominate, pubic, and ischium), softened by rickets, become deformed as they react to the pressures of weight from the upper body as well as from the frontal pull of muscles and tendons. These pressures produce a flattening of the pelvis from front to back, which can be exacerbated by lack of activity as well as increases in load-bearing (Loudon 1992, 1997; Ortner and Putchar 1981; Roberts and Manchester 1997). Female children who experience extreme cases of childhood rickets may have complications in childbirth, as the neonate's movement can be obstructed by the flattened pelvic shape, making it impossible to ascend the birth canal.

The impact of osteomalacia on adult bones is not as significant as in children, but it can still cause bowing of the legs and small changes in the pelvic bones if the condition is chronic and long-term. Osteomalacia can also cause an increase in issues related to osteoporosis (bone loss), such as increases in fractures. Chronic and long-term vitamin D deficiency ultimately will exhaust and compromise bone density, and can cause irreversible skeletal changes in the legs, pelvis, and even in the vertebral column (back) (see Figures 3.8 and 3.9).

For Victorian women, the impact of living with rickets on childhood growth and development, as well as the development of osteomalacia in young adulthood, clearly had a substantial effect on overall health across social classes. With the addition of cultural standards in which fasting and corset use were expected, as we discuss in further detail below, new patterns of ill-health, morbidity, and increases in mortality came to be seen as a normal part of daily life. Each of these factors had direct and lasting impacts on how women and female bodies were perceived, socially and biologically. All women in the Victorian period faced new social stressors that impacted their nutritional profiles, from not eating (if they were wealthy), or not having food (if they were poor). In addition, wealthy women were expected to maintain their pale facades, to present as white as possible, to ensure their status. The evolving race sciences supported an ideology that set middle- and upper-class bodies apart from supposedly less evolved, non-white bodies; this distinction, too, became a symbol of class difference. More elite white women chose to limit their exposure to sun as much as possible. For the working classes, exposure to sun was limited by long hours of work in the factories and the conditions of urban living, as well as from the darkened skies resulting from the smog of industrialization (Mosley 2001). The

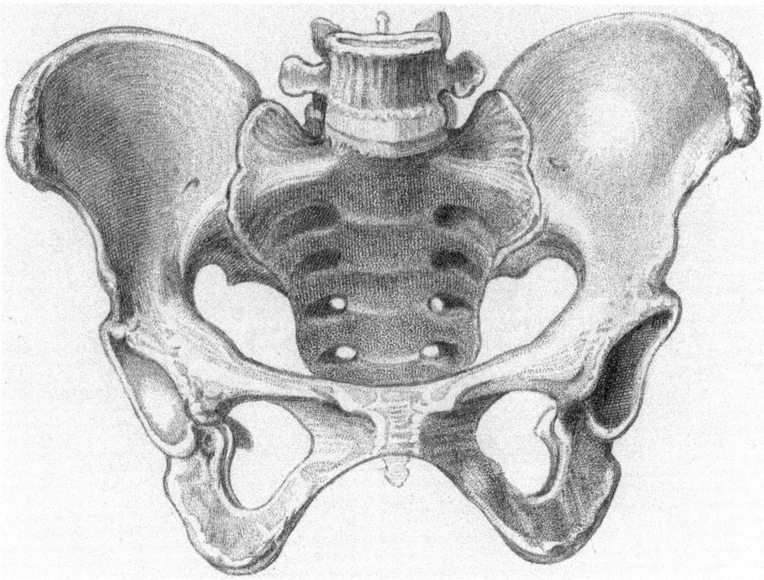

*Figure 3.8* Illustration of the normal female pelvis. Credit: Wellcome Collection. https://wellcomecollection.org/works/phva488j

overall reduction in stature for people of all classes during the Victorian era can be directly correlated to the social and environmental conditions of daily life, traces of which remain on the body and in the bones.

*Direct and Indirect Measures of Health*

Direct measures of stature (height) and rickets (morbidity) on the body reveal the biological consequences of nutritional deficiencies in the face of economic change. Similarly, the mortality profiles of females have been documented at higher rates during the Victorian era than any other time period (Mooney 2002). Victorian women's lives were affected by many factors which need to be considered as we examine the lived experience and mortality data. In the case of poor women, health issues reflect the social conditions to which they were subjected, in which a lack of access to nutritional resources was coupled with an increase in workload and the challenges of industrial labor. The health issues that can be identified in the case of well-to-do women are more closely linked to the social ideals of beauty and femininity expected of them.

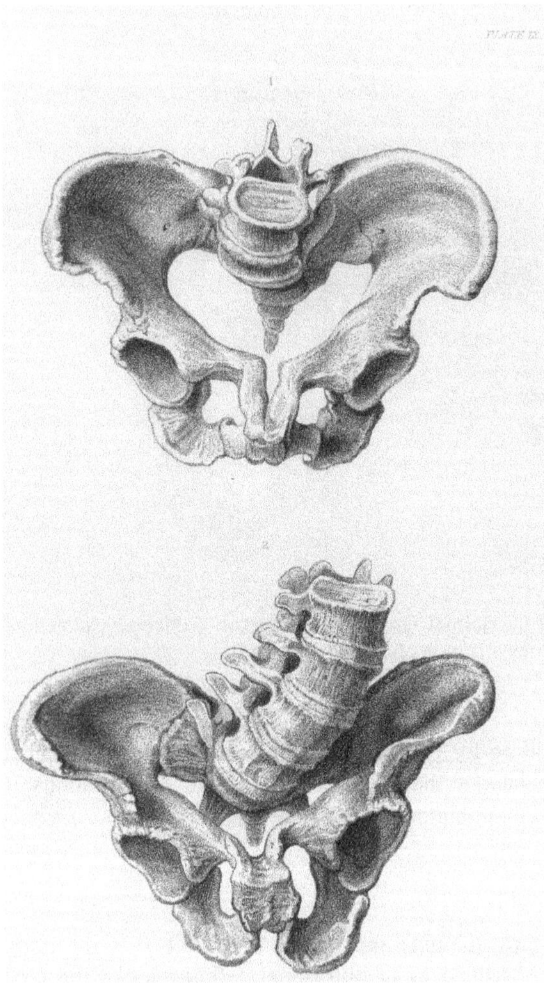

*Figure 3.9* Illustration of a deformed female pelvis from osteomalacia. Credit: Wellcome Collection. https://wellcomecollection.org/works/s5xdyq4s

Cultural expectations, shifting labor economies, and changing environments (quite literally, given the smog-filled skies from industrialization) form the backdrop for Victorians' lived experience. With these changes came great prosperity for some, scholars note, but there was also a wide gap between the rich and the poor—the "two nations" of nineteenth-century England.[1] These dynamics, combined with the effects of poor nutrition and changing realities around reproduction and birth (as we discuss in Chapter 4), had a synergistic effect on female quality and quantity of life.

Studies that focus on health and wellness during the industrial revolution reveal patterns of increases in female morbidity and mortality across class. Scholars have argued that these patterns reflect gender inequality, but it is difficult to distinguish between social and biological causes of gender differences in health and mortality (Harris 1998). Understanding the causes of female morbidity and mortality in Victorian England can shed light on the lived experiences of women, and it is here that we can begin to understand how the intersections of culture and biology impacted female health and wellness in this era.

For the middle and upper classes, the ideology of proper femininity, as set by Victorian codes of morality and behavior, required women to present themselves as delicate and unable to work hard. They were also required to maintain small bodies, which often meant they ate very little (Stacey 2002). Reduced food consumption resulted in nutritional deficiencies and smaller bodies, and was accompanied by bouts of fainting, and the appearance of being weaker—as indeed their bodies often were. Interestingly this behavior resulted in changes to the material culture of the era: fainting couches, smelling salts, and other items aimed to support the fragile woman became common household items, and are often seen as symbolic of Victorian culture as a whole.

Working-class women's social roles were almost diametrically opposed to those of the upper classes, as they were expected to work exceedingly hard for very little (Ehrenreich and English 1973). Working-class female bodies were believed by some to be more robust and therefore able to withstand the challenges of poor nutrition and ill health. Their lower economic status, however, often meant that they had limited access to food resources, and coupled with hard labor left them physically and nutritionally stressed. The economic and social reforms described earlier in this chapter went some way to addressing these issues, which became a matter of public health policy as the century progressed; but it was not until after the Victorian period that direct measures of health, more specifically maternal health, began to improve as a result of limits to working hours, improvements in industrial and housing conditions, as well as changes in medical practices (Komlos 1998).

## Shaping the Young Woman

While poor Victorian women's health was clearly compromised by the lack of resources, the moral codes and the ethics that governed women's behavior and appearance also had a profound effect on the female body. Codes of dress and fashion, in particular the ubiquitous use of corsets for all classes of women (Steele 2001) had a direct impact on their bodies and lives. Not only did the fashion dictate a "training" of the waist, with the goal of making the waistline as small as possible; advertisements and fashion magazines also underscored the importance of the period's signature hourglass silhouette, which required the woman to strive for thinness in order to obtain the smallest waist. In addition, the ability to refrain from eating reflected well on the individual woman, as she exerted the self-control embedded in the gender codes of the nineteenth century (Craton 2009).

### *Fasting Girls, Menstruation, and the Body Politic*

Several cases of "fasting girls" were highly publicized in Victorian medical and journalistic discourses; in these cases, young women (usually in early adolescence) would refrain from eating for long periods of time, whether for spiritual or physical reasons (Brumberg 1982, 1988; Gooldin 2003). Anorexia nervosa was first identified in England in 1873 by the physician William Withey Gull, who described its symptoms as "extreme emaciation, loss of appetite, amenorrhea, and restless activity" (Showalter 1985, 127) resulting from a "morbid mental state" (Gull 1874, cited in Showalter 1985). Whether or not they were diagnosed with anorexia nervosa or labeled "fasting girls" in the period's rhetoric, young women who limited their food intake were an extreme example of the period's emphasis on self-restraint (Showalter 1985; Silver 2002; Craton 2009).

Menarche, or the onset of the menstrual period, typically began for young women around age 12 or 13 (Steinbach 2017), although malnutrition might result in later onset of menses. Amenorrhea, or the temporary interruption of the menstrual cycle resulting in the loss of regular periods, was one result of self-starvation, and was of great concern to medical practitioners (Marland 2013). Victorian medical texts and popular advertisements alike exhorted women to attend to the regularity of their cycles, linking the proper circulation of menstrual blood to the proper functioning of the economy and society on a broader scale (Shuttleworth 1990). In this way, the female body came to stand in for the larger body politic, and young women were encouraged to consider a properly functioning menstrual cycle as critical to the reproductive health of the nation as a whole. Indeed, such discourses informed the young woman's sense of her role as a future mother to the citizens of the nation and the empire (Davin 1978), and underscored the importance of performing proper femininity in keeping with dominant cultural norms.

### *A Biocultural Case Study: Corsets and Costs*

Corsets in one form or another have been part of European culture for centuries, but the Victorian era marked a dramatic change in the ubiquitous use of the garment for all classes of women (Steele 2001). For Victorian era girls, corset use or waist training began around age nine and was facilitated by their mothers (Stone 2020), as noted by one mother in the society publication *Queen*:

> [W]ith my own daughters [...] [a]t the age of seven I had them fitted with stays without much bone and a flexible busk, and these were made to meet from top to bottom when laced, and so as not to exercise the least pressure round the chest and beneath the waist, and only a very slight pressure at the waist, just enough to show off the figure and give it a roundness.
>
> (as cited by Lord 1868, 167–168)

The corset was not just a fashion component for the nineteenth-century female body, but a symbol of proper womanhood as well (Summers 2001). While working-class women donned corsets that could accommodate their active work, embracing styles that laced in the front and could be loosened as needed, for middle- and upper-class women the introduction of tight-lacing, combined with the fashions of the era, dictated that the goal was to train the waist to be as small as possible. And given the ideological effects of the growing fashion and advertising industries, working-class women were not immune to the image requirements of the period (Summers 2001).

This model of tightly binding the body, combined with cultural restrictions on food consumption as well as physical activity and sun exposure, brought on a set of debilitating physical consequences that were joined with social discourses on the proper, and fragile, female form (Figure 3.10).

### *Biological Consequences*

A properly fitting corset is meant to target the waist, making it smaller than the "natural" or un-corseted waist. When a modern fitted corset is removed, the waist expands again, with few if any long-term effects on the body, although short-term effects can be observed, such as limitations to breathing capacity (Gau 1998; Steele 2001). Tight-lacing, or the practice of lacing the corset as tight as possible to train the waist to an even smaller size, had a markedly different effect on Victorian female bodies, particularly given the physiological and environmental conditions described above. When a corset

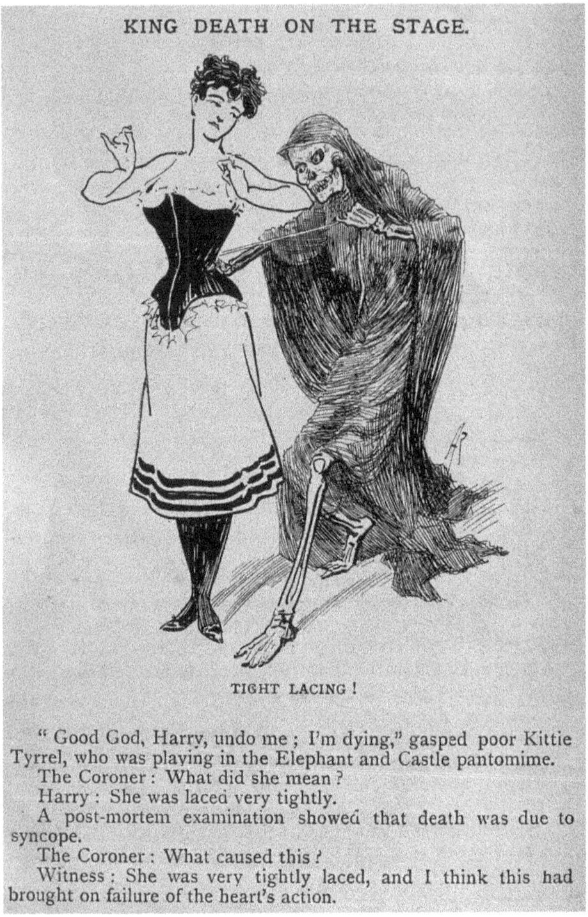
KING DEATH ON THE STAGE.
TIGHT LACING!
" Good God, Harry, undo me ; I'm dying," gasped poor Kittie Tyrrel, who was playing in the Elephant and Castle pantomime.
The Coroner : What did she mean ?
Harry : She was laced very tightly.
A post-mortem examination showed that death was due to syncope.
The Coroner : What caused this ?
Witness : She was very tightly laced, and I think this had brought on failure of the heart's action.

*Figure 3.10* The figure of a skeleton in a shroud is pulling the laces on a young girl's stays. Credit: Wellcome Collection. https://wellcomecollection.org/works/mvemyv2w

is contracted and tight-laced, the wearer's mobility is greatly decreased and the internal organs are displaced, shifting up into the thorax or down into the pelvic girdle and exerting pressure on the lungs or in the bowels and bladder (Figure 3.11).

This pressure results in shortness of breath (as the lungs cannot reach their full capacity), obstructed bowels, incontinence, and in some cases prolapsed uterus or bladder (Crutchfield 1897; Kunzel 2006). There are also skeletal responses, which include the squeezing in and up of the lower,

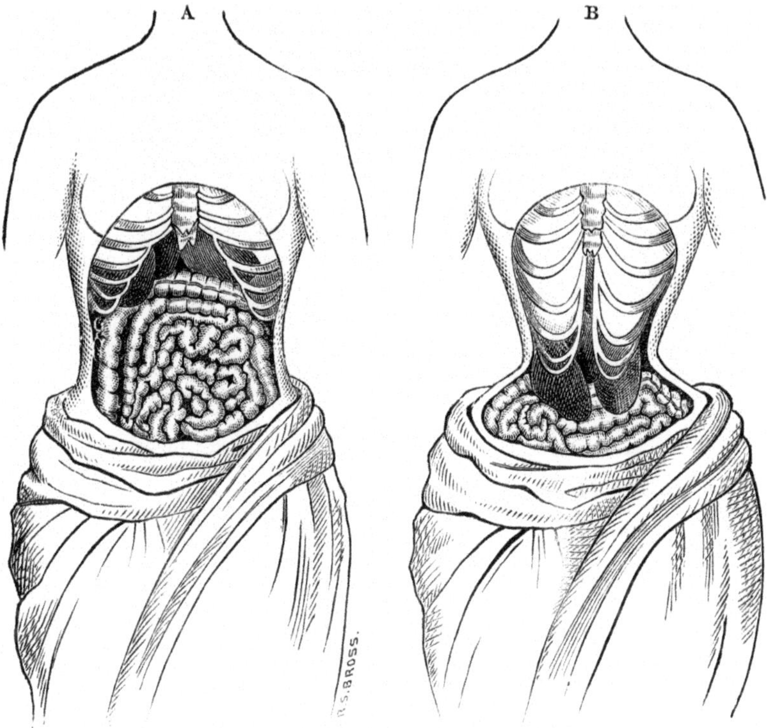


*Figure 3.11* Sketches from 1884 depicting what was believed to be the way the inside of the body looked when wearing a corset. A. natural position of internal organs; B. deformed by tight lacing, internal organs are compromised. Credit: Wikimedia Commons. https://en.wikipedia.org/wiki/Tightlacing#/media/File:ANatural_-_BTight_lacing.png

or floating, ribs, and a shifting of the vertebral articulation. When the corset is accompanied by a heavy dress, additional pressures are exerted on the pelvic girdle, pulling it down. The long-term effects of wearing a corset from childhood can involve the irreversible deformation of the pelvic girdle. When other health issues, such as rickets in childhood, were accompanied by corset use, these changes in the pelvic girdle were likely to result in complications in childbirth such as obstructed labor, dramatically increasing the risk of maternal morbidity and mortality (Stone 2009) (Figure 3.12).

In part as a result of the rickets epidemic for young children of all social status, the effects of tight-lacing can be seen in changes to the pelvic bones; bones softened by rickets were more spongy and malleable, resulting

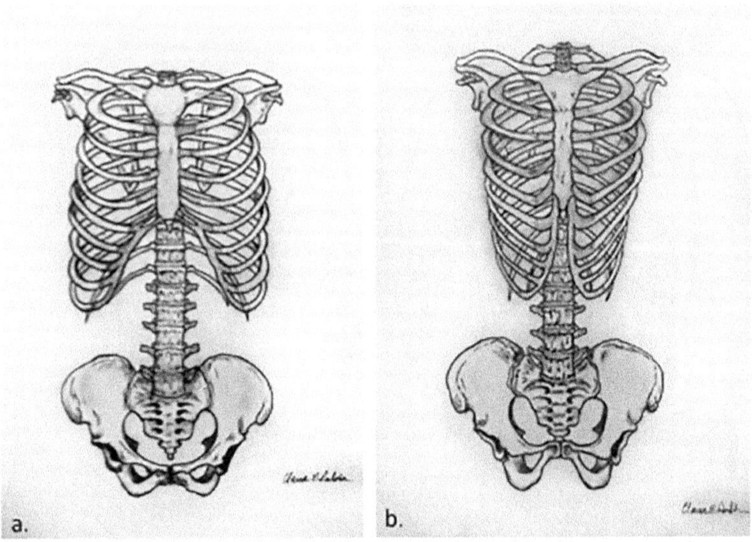


*Figure 3.12* A. Normal skeleton; B. skeleton showing the deformities from long-term corset wearing and rickets. Notice the changes in the ribs and in the pelvic girdle. (Artist, Claira Ralston)

in a waist that could become smaller and more pliable than ever before (Figure 3.13).

This pliability is noted from a young woman in a letter to the *Englishwoman's Domestic Magazine* in May 1867 (cited by both Lord 1868, 170 and Pichard 2005, 174):

> I was placed at the age of fifteen at a fashionable school in London, and there it was custom for the waists of the pupils to be reduced one inch per month until they were what the lady principal considered small enough. When I left school at seventeen, my waist measured only 13 inches, it having formerly been twenty-three inches in circumference.

Although scholars have noted that the "tight-lacing controversy" (as it was referred to in the press) and the actual extent of tight-lacing among Victorian girls and young women was exaggerated for the purposes of sensational and titillating journalistic effect (Beetham 1996), the practice of habitual corset use throughout a woman's waking hours and from girlhood through old age meant that the shape of the female body changed in identifiable ways.

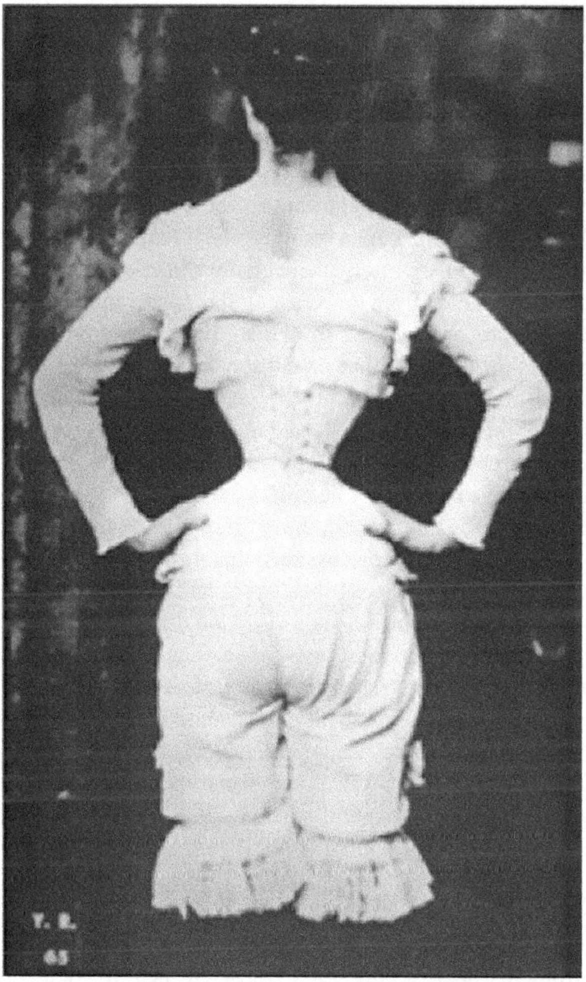

*Figure 3.13* Woman wearing a tight-laced corset, 1890. Credit: Victoria and Albert Museum, public domain. https://en.wikipedia.org/wiki/Tightlacing#/media/File:Wasp_waist.png

To sum up, the combined forces of biological indicators (metabolic disorders and changes to the position and pressures on the internal organs, and shape of the pelvis, ribs, and legs), social performance (corset use starting at a very early age, tight-lacing, and adherence to Victorian codes of femininity), and the changes brought on by the industrial revolution (reduced access to resources, diminished sunlight, increased/decreased labor) are all implicated in the increase in morbidity and mortality across classes for nineteenth-century women (Loudon 1997; Stone 2009). Health was stressed, and we can indirectly track and understand all these factors, utilizing archival documents, images, personal diaries, as well as written scholarship. But research into the direct consequences left on the body is constrained by a paucity of data. The bodies of women from the middle and upper classes were highly protected as a result of ideologies of mourning in the Victorian era (discussed in greater detail in Chapter 5). As a result, skeletal remains of white, middle- and upper-class women are rarely available for direct examination; instead, bodies that can be studied from this era are often traced to individuals who were poor, not white, or otherwise from marginalized groups.

Some recent scholarship (such as that of Gibson 2015) has attempted to explore the skeletal markers of corset use by examining medical and museum collections, but this work has neglected to consider that Victorian female bodies on display, or available for study in museums, rarely reflect the average person or the elite classes. While primary research on Victorian-era corseted skeletal remains is thin, we do know from other sources (vital statistics, personal narratives, medical discussions) that the practice of tight-lacing resulted in physical consequences that likely had morbid impacts (Gibson and Gibson 1903; O'Followell 1908; Loudon 1992, 1997). The Victorian woman's physical state, brought on by adherence to social scripts of status and proper femininity, both results in and reinforces the ideological discourse of middle- and upper-class white female bodies as fragile and pathologized. This body then becomes the representative "normal" female body: a body constrained from full physical and social mobility, which in the Victorian era became privileged over all others.

### *Fashion and Dress Reform*

In addition to the effects of corsetry and tight-lacing described in the previous section, women's dresses and skirts restricted their freedom of movement; despite dramatic changes to the silhouette over the course of the Victorian period, the consistency lies in the ways in which Victorian women's garments limited their mobility and therefore their physiological health (Figure 3.14). Although there were certainly differences in the types of garments worn depending on time of day, age, and profession, Victorian women were expected to conform to societal expectations for proper attire regardless of social status and class position.

Corset use varied significantly throughout the Victorian period, depending on changing fashions as well as on the life stage of the woman (Steele 2001; Summers 2001). Manufacturers marketed corsets specifically designed for

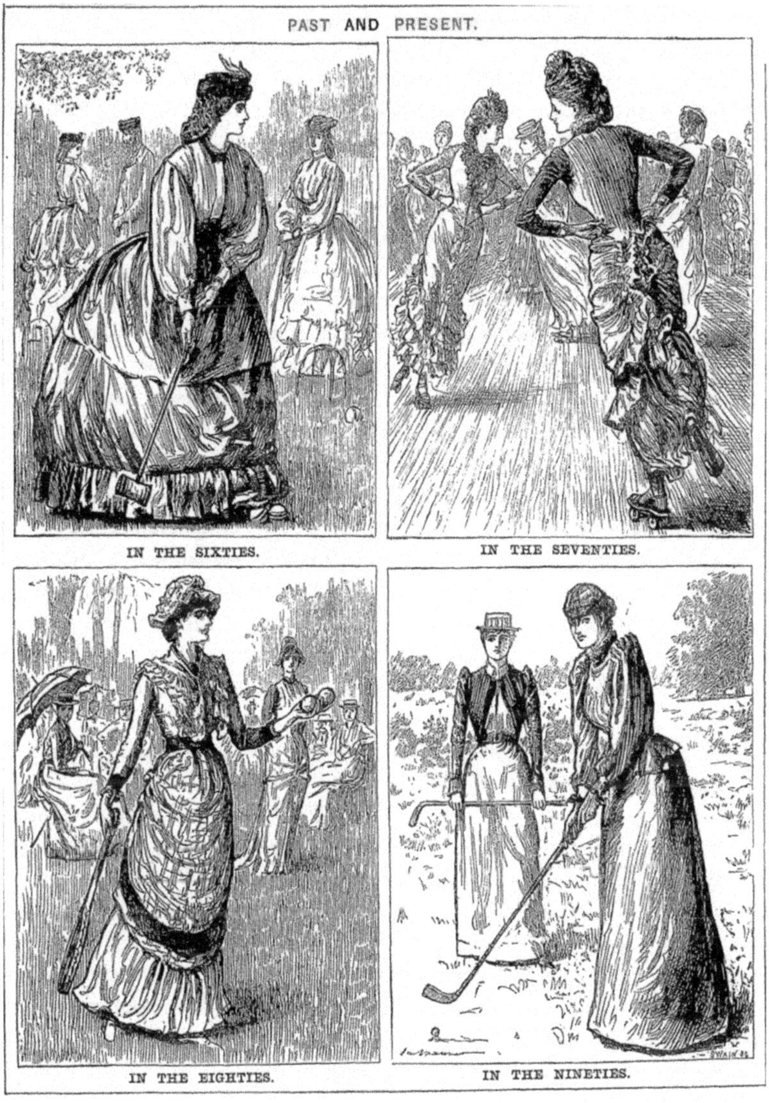


*Figure 3.14* "Past and Present." *Mr. Punch's Jubilee Number*, 18 July 1891. Vol. 101, p. 6. Public domain. Courtesy of Williston Library, Mount Holyoke College.

pregnancy and breastfeeding, as well as "orthopedic" and "electric" corsets (the latter so designated because electricity had been run through the metal stays, a dubious claim to technological advancement) (Steele 2001). The hourglass shape used throughout the century to accommodate the narrow waists and full skirts of the mid-Victorian era evolved to fit the bustle dresses of the 1870s and 1880s. In 1900 a French corsetière with a medical degree, Madame Inez Gâches-Sarraute, designed a "hygienic" straight-front corset intended to modify the negative health effects of the hourglass-shaped corset; but as Lynn Kutsche argues, this type of corset created an "S-bend" that pushed the shoulders and breasts forward, the abdomen and hips back, and put pressure on the pelvis, potentially leading to health complications (cited in Steele 2001, 84–85). Such complications were identified both at the time and in subsequent studies on historical re-enactors undergoing various physical tests while wearing corsets (Dickinson 1911; Gau 1998).

In addition to the corset, the shape and weight of skirts also had a burdensome effect on the female body. Prior to the 1840s, women would wear multiple petticoats to support the full skirts that became popular after the high, "Empire" waists of the first two decades of the nineteenth century. The advent of the crinoline (a petticoat stiffened with horsehair and whalebone) in the 1840s and the cage-crinoline (which modified the crinoline with steel hoops) in the 1850s made it possible for women to wear ever wider skirts, but constrained their movement, a phenomenon repeatedly satirized in *Punch* over the decades (Walkley 1985; Thomas 2004; Mitchell 2018) (Figure 3.15).

Other new dress designs and technologies similarly limited women's mobility. The invention of the bustle in the 1880s, which drew the fabric of the skirt around to the posterior, and the lengthy trains that accompanied this modification of the silhouette, made walking difficult; although the most elaborate examples were worn by wealthy and leisured women, the fashions nonetheless continued to constrict women's physical mobility. The "leg-of-mutton" sleeves fashionable in the 1880s and 1890s (so named after the French "gigot," or leg of lamb), shaped with full shoulders and narrow lower arms and wrists, severely limited women's arm movements; even the most common forms of shoulder seaming made it difficult for a woman to raise her arms above her head. Working women's garments were fitted less tightly to the body to enable greater mobility, but still were designed to avoid loose fabric that could get caught in machinery. Then as now, fashion had a trickle-down effect: the expensive, custom-made garments worn by the wealthiest women would be adapted by women of the middle and working classes into more affordable styles; however, the silhouette remained one that emphasized the wearer's fashionably thin waist in conformity with the sartorial expectations of the period.

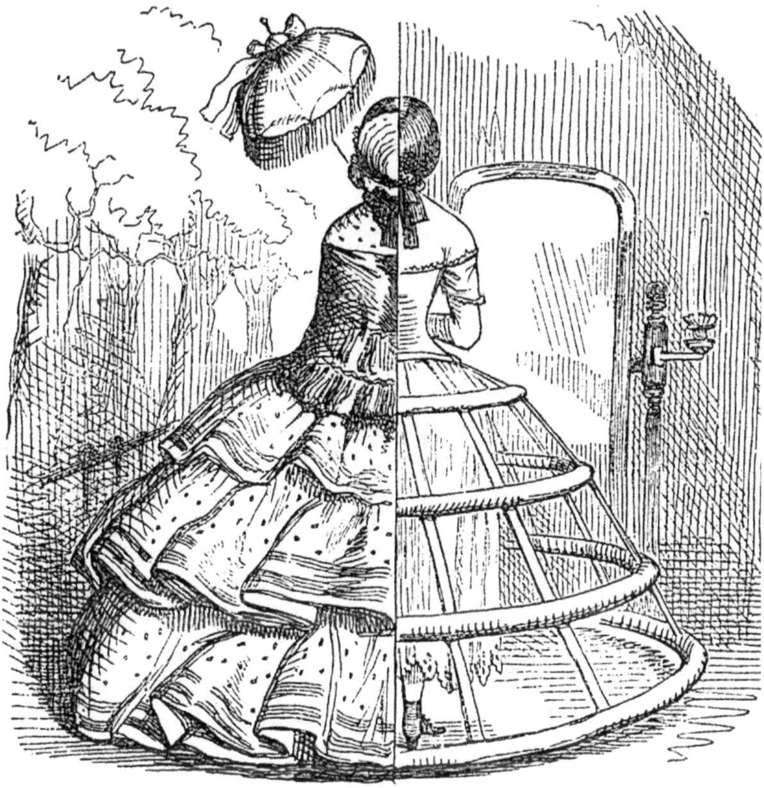

DRESS AND THE LADY.

*Figure 3.15* "Dress and the Lady." *Punch*, 23 August 1856. Vol. 31, p. 73. Public domain. Courtesy of Williston Library, Mount Holyoke College.

Gradually, as norms for feminine behavior changed, so too did clothing: not only the silhouette and the shape of the female body, but also the kinds of activities undertaken by women, with garments designed to accommodate them. The New Woman and her counterpart, the "New Girl," challenged the ideology of proper femininity in their pursuit of educational opportunities, sporting and leisure activities, and in forms of activity formerly labeled the province of men, such as smoking and bicycling (Mitchell 1995). In keeping with the logic of Social Darwinism, imperialism and national identity, middle-class girls were urged to undertake healthy but appropriate activities in order to keep their bodies strong for reproduction and motherhood. In the popular magazine *Girl's Own Paper*, "Medicus" (the pseudonym used by retired naval surgeon Gordon Stables) criticized the practice of tight-lacing and discouraged girls from using perfumed soaps and artificial beauty aids, instead encouraging readers to pursue wholesome activities like golf, walking, boating, fishing, and gardening. Cycling was considered acceptable as long as young women did not succumb to "cyclomania" (Moruzi 2012). Women needed special garments to undertake the newly fashionable leisure activity of bicycling, most notably a divided skirt or trousers; this new style corresponded with the increased popularity of masculine attire for women, in the form of bodice-and-skirt separates, suits, and eventually, the adoption of menswear-influenced style in the early twentieth century (Mitchell 2018) (Figure 3.16).

The turn toward clothing that permitted greater freedom of movement was inspired by earlier feminist critiques of fashion, among them the phenomenon of "bloomers," named after the United States women's rights activist Amelia Bloomer, who in turn publicized a costume designed by Elizabeth Smith Miller, which consisted of trousers to the ankle, with a short knee- or calf-length skirt (Figure 3.17).

In England, the Rational Dress Society, founded in 1881, formally opposed fashion that "deforms the figure, impedes the movements of the body, or in any way tends to injure the health" (The Rational Dress Society's *Gazette*, No. 4, January 1889, 1). In 1889, the Society established a Rational Dress Depot on Sloane Street in London, where women could purchase "underclothing, rational corsets and bodies, and divided skirts" at low cost. "Rational dress," also called "artistic" dress, was associated with the Aesthetic Movement in the 1870s and 1880s, which was influenced by the Pre-Raphaelite artists of the 1860s and whose proponents included William Morris, James McNeill Whistler, and Oscar Wilde (whose wife, Constance Wilde, edited the Rational Dress Society's *Gazette* in 1888 and 1889). In *The Art of Dress*, Mary Eliza Haweis (1879) argued for the relationship between "taste," beauty, and purpose in her critique of ornamentation in dress; likewise Florence Pomeroy (Viscountess Harberton), the President of the Rational Dress Society, argued for dress reform on the grounds of beauty, but also for reasons of health and safety, critiquing the use of tight bodices, clinging skirts, and impractical headwear. Lady Harberton conceded women's physical weakness as compared to men, but exhorted women to avoid exacerbating such weakness by the practice of

> literally so tying ourselves up in clothing that the muscles in some parts of the body dwindle until they become useless [and] the brain deteriorates from want of oxygen in the blood—brought about by the reduced

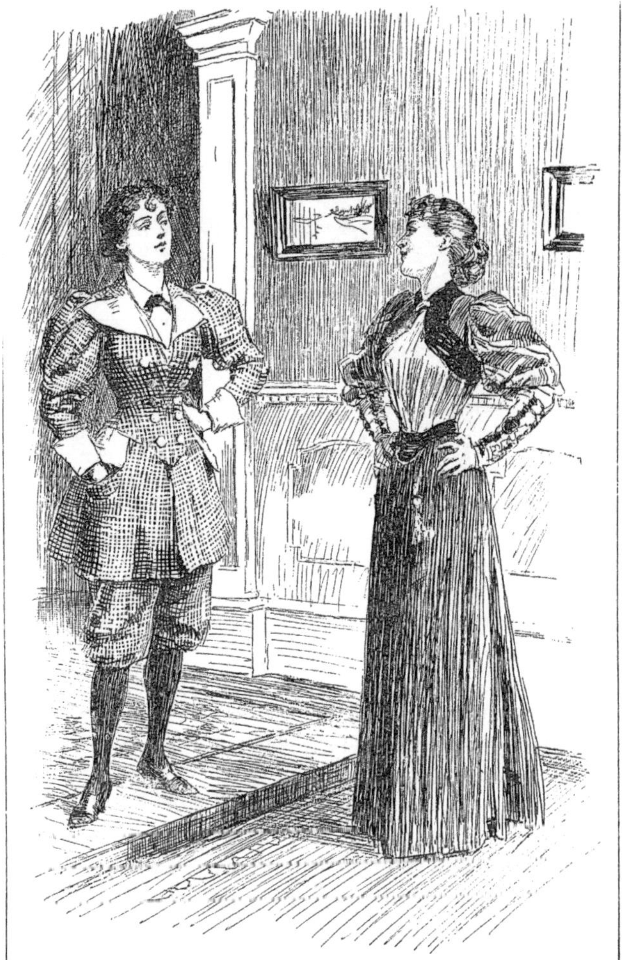

*Gertrude.* "My dear Jessie, what on earth is that Bicycle Suit for?"
*Jessie.* "Why, to wear, of course." *Gertrude.* "But you haven't got a Bicycle!"
*Jessie.* "No; but I've got a Sewing Machine!"

*Figure 3.16* "Bicycle suit." *Punch*, 12 January 1895. Vol. 108, p. 23. Public domain. Courtesy of Williston Library, Mount Holyoke College.

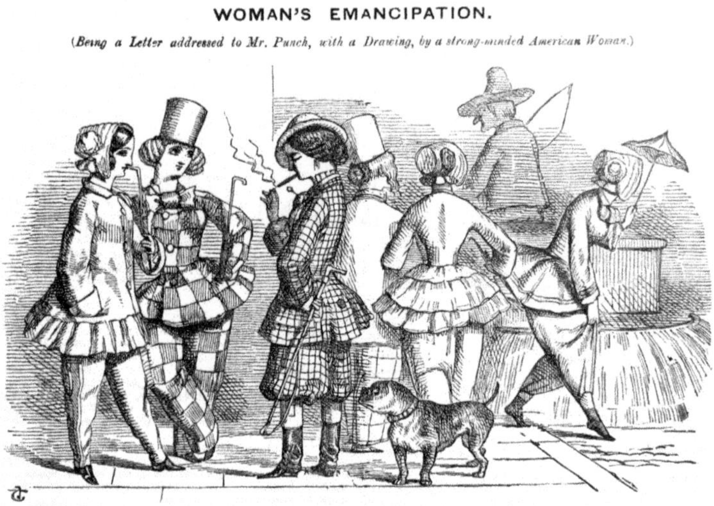
WOMAN'S EMANCIPATION.
(Being a Letter addressed to Mr. Punch, with a Drawing, by a strong-minded American Woman.)

*Figure 3.17* "Woman's Emancipation." *Punch,* 5 July 1851. Vol. 21, p. 3. Public domain. Courtesy of Amherst College Archives and Special Collections, Fitch/x/827 P969.

> breathing power inseparable from clothing so tight that the walls of the chest being unable to expand—the lungs cannot properly do their work of aerating the blood.
>
> (cited in Mitchell 2018, 81–82)

Although rational dress was not widely adopted in the era, and shorter hemlines, modified undergarments, and trousers for women were not embraced by the majority of the population until the twentieth century, these authors' arguments certainly led to a deeper understanding of the relationship between physical mobility and health, and eventually to a transformation in women's relationship to clothes.

In closing, it is important to reflect on the Victorians' understanding of gender, attire, and the body in the context of contemporary discussions of clothing and identity. Scholars of gender, queer theory, and transgender identity have illuminated the history of cross-gender identification and sartorial self-presentation, and such insights are helpful in order to contextualize the variety of gender identities that were associated with the term "woman" in the Victorian period. These identities included women who identified as feminine, masculine, or somewhere in between; women who wore menswear-inspired clothing and women who wore clothing associated with proper femininity; women who were heterosexual, lesbian, bisexual, and queer; married and unmarried women, spinsters, and sex workers; and women of all ages and classes (Marcus 2007; Liggins 2016). Current research into the range of gender identities embodied in Victorian culture enables a more nuanced understanding of girls' and young women's sexuality, physiology, and health in the nineteenth century.

## To Sum Up

- During the Industrial Revolution, health was influenced by economic shifts; across classes, there were measurable implications to health and wellness.
- Labor laws and debates over women's education engaged questions of women's health and preparedness to be in the workplace (as both children and adults) and to seek higher education.
- Class and health reverberated with the narrative of becoming a young woman: there was a powerful ideological emphasis on thinness and beauty as achieved through corsetry, tight-lacing, and fashion.
- Women were active in resisting these norms, both through the dress reform movement and various modes of questioning, critiquing, or reimagining gender.

## Questions to Consider

What are the ways we could learn more about stature (height) for Victorian women across the classes to understand the direct impact of nutritional deficiencies that they faced?

## Note

1 Benjamin Disraeli, who served twice as Prime Minister (in 1868 and 1874–1880), published a novel entitled *Sybil, or the Two Nations*, in 1845. His work was inspired in part by the 1838 People's Charter and the Chartist Movement, which advocated for universal male suffrage and electoral reform, and the economic depression leading to a series of famines in the "Hungry Forties." The gulf between the rich and the poor formed the basis for social problem novels by Charles Dickens, Elizabeth Gaskell, and other authors addressing the "Condition of England" in the 1840s.

## References

### *Primary Sources*

Barrett Browning, Elizabeth. 1857. *Aurora Leigh*. Edited with an introduction by Kerry McSweeney. Oxford: Oxford World's Classics, 1998.

Chadwick, Edwin Hammond. 1842. *Report on the Sanitary Condition of the Labouring Population of Great Britain*. House of Commons Sessional Paper, Vol. XXVI. https://www.parliament.uk/about/living-heritage/transformingsociety/livinglearning/coll-9-health1/health-02/. Accessed 20 September 2019.

Clarke, Edward. 1873. *Sex in Education: A Fair Chance for the Girls*. Boston, MA: James R. Osgood and Co.

Crutchfield, E.L. 1897. "Some Ill Effects of the Corset." *Gaillard's Medical Journal* 67 (July): 37–14.

Davies, Emily. 1866. *The Higher Education of Women*. London: Alexander Strahan.

Disraeli, Benjamin. 1845. *Sybil, Or The Two Nations*. Edited with an introduction by Nicholas Shrimpton. Oxford: Oxford World's Classics, 2017.

Ellis, Sarah Stickney. 1839. *The Women of England, Their Social Duties, and Domestic Habits*. New York: D. Appleton and Co.

Engels, Friedrich. 1845; trans. 1892. *The Condition of the Working Class in England*. London: G. Allen and Unwin, Ltd.

Garrett Anderson, Elizabeth. 1874. "Sex in Mind and Education: A Reply." *Fortnightly Review* 15 (May): 582–594.

Gibson, J.W., and J. W. Gibson. 1903. "Illus." In *Golden Thoughts on Chastity and Procreation, Including Heredity, Prenatal Influences, etc.: Sensible Hints and Wholesome Advice for Maiden and Young Man, Wife and Husband, Mother and Father*, 106–108. Naperville, IL: J. L. Nichols.

Gull, William Withey. 1874. "Anorexia Nervosa." *Transactions of the Clinical Society of London* 7: 22–28.

Haweis, H. R. (Mary Eliza). 1879. *The Art of Dress*. London: Chatto and Windus.

Hotchkiss, Louise S. 1873. "Corsets, Versus Brains." *Cambridge Chronicle* XXVIII (10) (8 March): 1.

Lord, William Barry. 1868. *The Corset and the Crinoline: A Book of Modes and Costumes, from Remote Periods to the Present Time*. London: Ward, Lock, and Tyler.

Maudsley, Henry. 1874. "Sex in Mind and in Education." *Fortnightly Review* 15 (April): 466–483.

Mayhew, Henry. 1851–1852. *London Labour and the London Poor*. Edited with an introduction by Victor Neuberg. London/New York: Penguin, 1985.

Mitchell, Silas Weir. 1871. *Wear and Tear, or Hints for the Overworked*. Philadelphia, PA: J. B. Lippincott and Co.

O'Followell, Ludovic. 1908. "Fig. 31. Radiographie du corset Ligne (devant)." In *Le Corset*. Maloine. http://commons.wikimedia.org/wiki/File:Radiographie du corset Ligne (devant).jpg (accessed through Wikimedia, 01.03.12).

Oliver, Thomas. 1902. *Dangerous Trades: The Historical, Social, and Legal Aspects of Industrial Occupations as Affecting Health, by a Number of Experts*. London: J. Murray.

### *Secondary Sources*

Beetham, Margaret. 1996. *A Magazine of Her Own? Domesticity and Desire in the Woman's Magazine, 1800–1914*. London: Routledge.

Brickley, Megan, and Rachel Ives. 2008. *The Bioarchaeology of Metabolic Bone Disease*. Oxford: Academic Press.

Brumberg, Joan Jacobs. 1982. "Chlorotic girls, 1870–1920: A Historical Perspective on Female Adolescence." *Child Development* 53: 1468–1477.

Brumberg, Joan Jacobs. 1988. *Fasting Girls: The Emergence of Anorexia Nervosa as a Modern Disease*. Cambridge, MA: Harvard University Press.

Caine, Barbara. 1992. *Victorian Feminists*. Oxford: Oxford University Press.

Cameron, Noel, and Ellen W. Demerath. 2002. "Critical Periods in Human Growth and Their Relationship to Diseases of Aging." *American Journal of Physical Anthropology: The Official Publication of the American Association of Physical Anthropologists* 119 (S35): 159–184.

Craton, Lillian. 2009. *The Victorian Freak Show: The Significance of Disability and Physical Differences in 19th-Century Fiction*. Amherst, NY: Cambria Press.

Davin, Anna. 1978. "Imperialism and Motherhood." *History Workshop Journal* 5 (1): 9–66.

Danforth, Marie E., Kristrina Shuler, and Jeffrey Auerbach. 2011. "Challenges in Approaches to Skeletal Stature Estimation: An Example from Prehistoric Eastern Mississippi/Western Alabama." *American Journal of Physical Anthropology* 144 (S52): 120.

DeWitte, Sharon N., Gail Hughes-Morey, Jelena Bekvalac, and Jordan Karsten. 2016. "Wealth, Health and Frailty in Industrial-Era London." *Annals of Human Biology* 43 (3): 241–254.

Dickinson, Robert L. 1911. "Toleration of the Corset: Prescribing Where One Cannot Proscribe." *American Journal of Obstetrics and Gynecology* 63: 1023–1058.

Dobbie, B.M. Willmott. 1982. "An Attempt to Estimate the True Rate of Maternal Mortality, Sixteenth to Eighteenth Centuries." *Medical History* 26 (1): 79–90.

Dyhouse, Carol. 1981. *Girls Growing Up in Late Victorian and Edwardian England*. London: Routledge and Kegan Paul.

Ehrenreich, Barbara, and Deirdre English. 1973. *Witches, Midwives, and Nurses: A History of Women Healers*. New York: Feminist Press.

Emsley, John. 2004. *The 13th Element: The Sordid Tale of Murder, Fire, and Phosphorous*. New York: John Wiley and Sons.

Fletcher, Anthony. 2008. *Growing Up in England: The Experience of Childhood, 1600–1914*. New Haven, CT: Yale University Press.

Gau, Colleen Ruby. 1998. "Historic Medical Perspectives of Corseting and Two Physiologic Studies with Reenactors." PhD diss., Iowa State University. *Retrospective Theses and Dissertations*. 11922. https://lib.dr.iastate.edu/rtd/11922.

Gibbs, Denis. 1994. "Rickets and the Crippled Child: An Historical Perspective." *Journal of the Royal Society of Medicine* 87 (12): 729.

Gibson, Rebecca. 2015. "Effects of Long Term Corseting on the Female Skeleton: A Preliminary Morphological Examination." *Nexus*: *The Canadian Student Journal of Anthropology* 23 (2): 45–60.

Gooldin, Sigal. 2003. "Fasting Women, Living Skeletons, and Hunger Artists: Spectacles of Body and Miracles at the Turn of a Century." *Body & Society* 9 (2): 27–53.

Gordon, Peter, and David Doughan. 2001. *Dictionary of British Women's Organisations, 1825–1960*. London: Woburn Press.
Gowland, Rebecca. 2018. "'A Mass of Crooked Alphabets': The Construction and Othering of Working-Class Bodies in Industrial England." In *Bioarchaeological Analyses and Bodies: New Ways of Knowing Anatomical and Archaeological Skeletal Collections*, edited by Pamela K. Stone, 147–163. Cham, Switzerland: Springer.
Gowland, Rebecca L., A. C. Caffell, Sophie Newman, Alysa Levene, and Malin Holst. 2018. "Broken Childhoods: Rural and Urban Non-Adult Health During the Industrial Revolution in Northern England (Eighteenth-Nineteenth Centuries)." *Bioarchaeology International* 2 (1): 44–62.
Greenlees, Janet. 2007. *Female Labour Power: Women Workers' Influence on Business Practices in the British and American Cotton Industries, 1780–1860*. Aldershot, England: Ashgate.
Hardy, Anne. 1992. "Rickets and the Rest: Child-Care, Diet and the Infectious Children's Diseases, 1850–1914." *Social History of Medicine* 5 (3): 389–412.
Harris, Bernard. 1998. "Gender, Height and Mortality in Nineteenth- and Twentieth-Century Britain: Some Preliminary Reflections." In *The Biological Standard of Living in Comparative Perspective*, edited by John Komlos and Joerg Baten, 413–448. Stuttgart: Franz Steiner Verlag.
Harris, Bernard. 2008. "Gender, Health, and Welfare in England and Wales Since Industrialisation." In *Research in Economic History*, edited by Alexander J. Field, Gregory Clark, William A. Sundstrom, 157–204. Bingley: Emerald Group Publishing Limited.
Harrison, Barbara. 1996. *Not Only the 'Dangerous Trades': Women's Work and Health in Britain, 1880–1914*. London: Taylor and Francis.
Higgs, Edward. 1983. "Domestic Servants and Households in Victorian England". *Social History* 8 (2): 201–210.
Horrell, Sarah, Jane Humphries, and Hans-Joachim Voth. 1998. "Stature and Relative Deprivation: Fatherless Children in Early Industrial Britain." *Continuity and Change* 13 (1): 73–115.
Jordan, Ellen. 1999. *The Women's Movement and Women's Employment in Nineteenth-Century Britain*. London/New York: Routledge.
Jowitt, J. A., and A. J. McIvor, eds. 1988. *Employers and Labour in the English Textile Industries, 1850–1939*. London/New York: Routledge.
Komlos, John. 1993. "The Secular Trend in the Biological Standard of Living in the United Kingdom, 1730–1860." *The Economic History Review* 46 (1): 115–144.
Komlos, John. 1998. "Shrinking in a Growing Economy? The Mystery of Physical Stature During the Industrial Revolution." *The Journal of Economic History* 58 (3): 779–802.
Kunzel, David. 2006. *Fashion & Fetishism: Corsets, Tight-Lacing and Other Forms of Body-Sculpture*. Cheltenham: The History Press.
Lacey, Candida Ann, ed. 2001. *Barbara Leigh Smith Bodichon and the Langham Place Group*. Vol. III of the Women's Source Library. London: Routledge.

Levine-Clark, Marjorie. 2004. *Beyond the Reproductive Body: The Politics of Women's Health and Work in Early Victorian England*. Columbus, OH: The Ohio State University Press.

Lewis, Mary E. 2002. "Impact of Industrialization: Comparative Study of Child Health in Four Sites from Medieval and Postmedieval England (AD 850–1859)." *American Journal of Physical Anthropology: The Official Publication of the American Association of Physical Anthropologists* 119 (3): 211–223.

Liggins, Emma. 2016. *Odd Women? Spinsters, Lesbians and Widows in British Women's Fiction, 1850s–1930s*. Manchester: Manchester University Press.

Lips, P. 2006. "Vitamin D Physiology." *Progress in Biophysics and Molecular Biology* 92 (1): 4–8.

Loudon, Irvine. 1992. *Death in Childbirth: An International Study of Maternal Care and Maternal Mortality, 1800–1950*. Oxford: Oxford University Press.

Loudon, Irvine. 1997. *Western Medicine: An Illustrated History*. Oxford: Oxford University Press.

Malone, Carolyn. 2003. *Women's Bodies and Dangerous Trades in England, 1880–1914*. London: Royal Historical Society; Woodbridge, UK/New York: Boydell Press.

Marcus, Sharon. 2007. *Between Women: Friendship, Desire, and Marriage in Victorian England*. Princeton, NJ: Princeton University Press.

Marland, Hilary. 2013. *Health and Girlhood in Britain, 1874–1920*. Houndmsills, Basingstoke, Hampshire: Palgrave Macmillan.

Mathews David, Alison. 2015. *Fashion Victims: The Dangers of Dress Past and Present*. London/New York: Bloomsbury.

Mays, Simon, Megan Brickley, and Rachel Ives. 2008. "Growth in an English Population from the Industrial Revolution." *American Journal of Physical Anthropology: The Official Publication of the American Association of Physical Anthropologists* 136 (1): 85–92.

McDermid, Jane. 2012. *The Schooling of Girls in Britain and Ireland, 1800–1914*. London/New York: Routledge.

Mitchell, Rebecca, ed. 2018. *Fashioning the Victorians: A Critical Sourcebook*. London: Bloomsbury.

Mitchell, Sally. 1995. *The New Girl: Girls' Culture in England, 1880–1915*. New York: Columbia University Press.

Mooney, Graham. 2002. "Shifting Sex Differentials in Mortality During Urban Epidemiological Transition: The Case of Victorian London." *International Journal of Population Geography* 8 (1): 17–47.

Moruzi, Kristine. 2012. *Constructing Girlhood Through the Periodical Press, 1850–1915*. Farnham, Surrey: Ashgate.

Mosley, Stephen. 2001. *The Chimney of the World: A History of Smoke Pollution in Victorian and Edwardian Manchester*. Cambridge: White Horse Press.

Nardinelli, Clark. 1980. "Child Labor and the Factory Acts." *The Journal of Economic History* 40 (4): 739–755.

Nash, Linda. 2015. "Toxic Century: The Origins of 'Environmental Health.'" Published in French as "Un siècle toxique. Les origines de la 'santé environnementale.'" *Histoire de Sciences et des Savoirs*, v. 3, edited by Dominique Pestre and Christophe Bonneuil, 144–165. Paris: Le Seuil/Palgrave.

Nelson, Claudia. 1999. "Growing Up: Childhood." In *A Companion to Victorian Literature and Culture*, edited by Herbert F. Tucker, 67–81. Malden, MA: Blackwell Publishers.

Newman, Sophie L., and Rebecca L. Gowland. 2016. "Dedicated Followers of Fashion? Bioarchaeological Perspectives on Socio-economic Status, Inequality, and Health in Urban Children from the Industrial Revolution (18th–19th C)." *International Journal of Osteoarchaeology* 27 (2): 217–229.

Nitsch, Erika K., Louise T. Humphrey, and Robert E. M. Hedges. 2011. "Using Stable Isotope Analysis to Examine the Effect of Economic Change on Breastfeeding Practices in Spitalfields, London, UK." *American Journal of Physical Anthropology* 146 (4): 619–628.

Ortner, Donald J., and Walter G. J. Putschar. 1981. *Identification of Pathological Conditions in Human Skeletal Remains*. Washington, DC: Smithsonian Institution Press.

Pichard, Liza. 2005. *Victorian London: The Tale of a City 1840–1870*. Houndsmills, Basingstoke, Hampshire, and London: Macmillan.

Pollock, Richard A., Ted W. Brown Jr., and David M. Rubin. 2015. "'Phossy Jaw' and 'Bis-Phossy Jaw' of the 19th and the 21st Centuries: The Diuturnity of John Walker and the Friction Match." *Craniomaxillofacial Trauma & Reconstruction* 8 (3): 262–270.

Raw, Louise. 2011. *Striking a Light: The Bryant and May Matchwomen and Their Place in History*. London: Continuum.

Roberts, Charlotte A., Anwen Caffell, Kori L. Filipek-Ogden, Rebecca Gowland, and Tina Jakob. 2016. "'Til Poison Phosphorous Brought Them Death': A Potentially Occupationally-Related Disease in a Post-Medieval Skeleton from North-East England." *International Journal of Paleopathology* 13: 39–48.

Roberts, Charlotte, and Keith Manchester. 1997. *The Archaeology of Disease*. 2nd ed. Ithaca, NY: Cornell University Press.

Satre, Lowell J. 1982. *After the Match Girls' Strike: Bryant and May in the 1890s*. Bloomington, IN: Indiana University Press.

Sanders, Lise Shapiro (2015). "'Equal Laws Based upon an Equal Standard': The Garrett Sisters, the Contagious Diseases Acts, and the Sexual Politics of Victorian and Edwardian Feminism Revisited." *Women's History Review* 24 (3): 389–409.

Showalter, Elaine. 1985. *The Female Malady: Women, Madness, and English Culture, 1830–1980*. New York: Penguin.

Shuttleworth, Sally. 1990. "Female Circulation: Medical Discourse and Popular Advertising in the Mid-Victorian Era." In *Body/Politics: Women and the Discourses of Science*, edited by Mary Jacobus, Evelyn Fox Keller, and Sally Shuttleworth, 47–68. New York: Routledge.

Silver, Anna Krugovoy. 2002. *Victorian Literature and the Anorexic Body*. Cambridge/New York: Cambridge University Press.

Stacey, Michelle. 2002. *The Fasting Girl: A True Victorian Medical Mystery*. New York: Jeremy P. Tarcher.

Steckel, Richard H. 1995. "Stature and the Standard of Living." *Journal of Economic Literature* 33 (4): 1903–1940.

Steele, Valerie. 2001. *The Corset: A Cultural History*. New Haven, CT: Yale University Press.

Steinbach, Susie. 2004. *Women in England 1760–1914: A Social History*. New York: Palgrave Macmillan.

Steinbach, Susie L. 2012; 2nd ed. 2017. *Understanding the Victorians: Politics, Culture and Society in Nineteenth-Century Britain*. London/New York: Routledge.

Stone, Pamela K. 2009. "A History of Western Medicine, Labor, and Birth." In *Childbirth Across Cultures: Ideas and Practices of Pregnancy, Birth, and the Postpartum*, edited by Helaine Selin and Pamela K. Stone, 41–53. Dordrecht: Springer.

Stone, Pamela K. 2020. "Bound to Please: The Shaping of Female Beauty, Gender Theory, Structural Violence, and Bioarchaeological Investigations." In *Purposeful Pain: The Bioarchaeology of Intentional Suffering*, edited by Susan Sheridan, Susan Guise and Lesley Gregoricka, 39–62. Cham, Switzerland: Springer Nature.

Summers, Leigh. 2001. *Bound to Please: A History of the Victorian Corse*t. Oxford: Berg.

Teleky, Ludwig. 1948. *History of Factory and Mine Hygiene*. New York: Columbia University Press, 1948.

Theobald, H. E. 2005. "Dietary Calcium and Health." *Nutrition Bulletin* 30 (3): 237–277.

Thomas, Julia. 2004. *Pictorial Victorians: The Inscription of Values in Word and Image*. Athens, OH: Ohio University Press.

Walkley, Christina. 1985. *The Way to Wear'em: 150 Years of Punch on Fashion*. London: P. Owen.

Wells, Jonathan C. K., Jeremy M. DeSilva, and Jay T. Stock. 2012. "The Obstetric Dilemma: An Ancient Game of Russian Roulette, or a Variable Dilemma Sensitive to Ecology?" *American Journal of Physical Anthropology* 149 (S55): 40–71.

Whorton, James C. 2010. *The Arsenic Century: How Victorian Britain Was Poisoned at Home, Work, and Play*. Oxford: Oxford University Press.


### *Online Resources*


Mayo Clinic. 2019. "Rickets – Symptoms and Causes." Mayo Foundation for Medical Education and Research (MFMER): https:/www.mayoclinic.org/diseases-conditions/rickets/symptoms-causes/syc-20351943. Accessed 5 September 2019.

1833 Factory Act: https://www.parliament.uk/about/living-heritage/transforming society/livinglearning/19thcentury/overview/factoryact/. Accessed 14 June 2019.

Rational Dress Society. The Rational Dress Society's *Gazette* (January 1889). Held by the British Library, shelfmark 1866.b.9.(10.): https://www.bl.uk/collection-items/the-rational-dress-societys-gazette. Accessed 31 August 2019.

# 4 The Good Mother and the Proper Wife

## Marriage, Pregnancy, and Motherhood

### Introduction

This chapter explores the life stage central to the ideology of proper Victorian womanhood, examining how social constructions of femininity are intimately woven into the physicality of marriage and motherhood. In addition, this is the stage of life that garners the most attention from the developing fields of science and medicine (particularly obstetrics and gynaecology), as it represents the apex of reproductive capacity. In this chapter we examine not only the medical discourses surrounding female bodily experience, but also the legal frameworks that came under increasing scrutiny as women activists strove to reform the laws affecting women's lives. We look to literary texts not for evidence of women's lived experience, but rather as evidence of the ways in which literature both reflects and produces cultural narratives around proper femininity in the Victorian era. We also examine cultural discourses around women who deviated from prescribed paths, exploring how the decision to remain single may have helped women to express resistance to the powerful ideology of marriage and motherhood throughout this period.

We begin by considering how women's bodily experience within marriage was scripted through constructions of the family and the home that in turn relied on the image of the "angel in the house" and the myth of separate spheres. We then turn to a discussion of legislative changes that affected the lives of married women and mothers, particularly with respect to issues of marital conflict (separation and divorce), women's property, and child custody. As the nineteenth century progressed a number of activist and reform efforts enabled women (and men) to call for improvements in child welfare, girls' and women's working conditions, and education. Early feminist networks provided a forum for women to address these issues and, as the suffrage movement advanced in the latter half of the century, to press for the vote as a symbol of women's demand for citizenship and equal treatment under the law. We follow this discussion with an analysis of issues affecting women who, by choice or necessity, lived outside of the norms of marriage: we address the treatment of single mothers in the Victorian era, and explore the figures of the spinster, the "fallen woman," and the prostitute. Debates over the sexual double standard and the management of sexually transmitted diseases, as well as the issue of family planning and access to birth control, were central to the ways in which women's bodily autonomy and agency were conceived. We conclude the chapter with a discussion of Victorian perspectives on pregnancy and childbirth, breastfeeding, and childrearing, as a window into the lived experiences of mothers over the course of their reproductive years.

## Marriage and the Construction of the Family

### *The Angel in the House and the Myth of Separate Spheres*

The Victorian doctrine of separate spheres was a construction, more myth than reality, and masked the varied involvement of women in public life in the eighteenth and nineteenth centuries (Vickery 1993). Nevertheless, the notion of the home as a feminine realm had its foundations in a number of Victorian texts that strove to delineate the ideal characteristics of wives and mothers. Coventry Patmore's poem *The Angel in the House* (published in parts between 1854 and 1862) is often cited as a key text in the ideological production of proper femininity in the Victorian era. Patmore's poem elaborates the qualities of the ideal wife—dignity, modesty, grace, and charm—while also underscoring that wives find their reward in their devotion and submission to their husbands' wishes: "Man must be pleased; but him to please / Is woman's pleasure" (Patmore, Book I, Canto IX, ll. 1–2). In a similar vein, John Ruskin, well known as a leading Victorian critic of art and architecture, published a pair of essays in his 1865 book *Sesame and Lilies* entitled "Of Kings' Treasuries" and "Of Queens' Gardens," the latter emphasizing women's role as guardians of the home and hearth and especially their moral and spiritual influence over their husbands and children:

> The man's power is active, progressive, defensive. He is eminently the doer, the creator, the discoverer, the defender. His intellect is for speculation and invention; his energy for adventure, for war, and for conquest, wherever war is just, wherever conquest necessary. But the woman's power is for rule, not for battle—and her intellect is not for invention or creation, but for sweet ordering, arrangement, and

> decision. […] This is the true nature of home—it is the place of Peace; the shelter, not only from all injury, but from all terror, doubt, and division.
>
> (Ruskin 1865, 77, emphasis in original)

Ruskin's phrasing makes clear the distinction here drawn between the two gendered spheres, and underscores the characteristics of the ideal woman who ministers to the home and family: "She must be enduringly, incorruptibly good; instinctively, infallibly wise—wise, not for self-development, but for self-renunciation: wise, not that she may set herself above her husband, but that she may never fail from his side: wise, not with the narrowness of insolent and loveless pride" (Ruskin 1865, 78). This focus on women's domestic role precisely at the time when more and more women were embarking on careers in higher education and the professions reveals not only the power of such ideological and social frameworks, but also the realities they strove to counteract (Mitchell 1996). Importantly, too, relegating middle- and upper-class women to the home had significant economic, social, and cultural effects, and also played a role in their physical and mental health (particularly in the frequent diagnosis of hysteria), as we discuss at greater length below.

In short, Victorian men and women grappled with an ideology of gender difference that saw marriage and motherhood as the endpoint of women's lives. This was a view that was central to the focus of science, as reproduction was constitutive to Victorian understandings of sexual difference, and informed the social production of gender. As a result, a number of approaches to women's education, particularly in what was termed "domestic economy," were framed in terms of their impact on reproduction and the ways that education might disrupt women's role as wives and mothers.

Exceptions to this narrative of married women as sole domestic managers and guardians of the home existed. For the titled and landed classes, the caretaking duties associated with the ideology of motherhood—particularly infant and child care, and education—were taken over by nurses, maids, tutors and governesses, and schoolteachers when children attended school outside the home. Since women were frequently employed in these positions, this resulted in a shift to paid domestic labor rather than unpaid labor on the part of the wife and mother. Not all of these positions required training, but those that did, such as teaching and nursing, were often seen as most appropriate for unmarried women without children ("spinsters," in the period's rhetoric)—further underscoring education's perceived inverse relationship to reproductive fertility. Married women in the professions typically employed servants themselves (often considered a mark of class that distinguished the upper and middle classes from the working classes and the poor), and the increasing number of women employed in white-collar jobs in the service sector might spend a longer period of time working before marriage, as the so-called "marriage bar" (prohibiting women from marrying while employed as teachers, for example) was not abolished until the Sex Disqualification Removal Act of 1919. Working- and middle-class women were subject to what feminists then and now have called the "second shift," working at paid employment during the day and tending to home, husband, and children in the evening (Hamilton 1909; Hochschild and Machung 1989; Steinbach 2004). The economic disparities between married women of different classes—and the discrimination against all married women in the laws relating to suffrage, property, and parenthood—led to changes to the laws affecting marriage, divorce, and child custody that occurred throughout the Victorian period (Stetson 1982; Holcombe 1983; Perkin 1989; Phegley 2012).

### *Legislating Lives and Property: Marriage, Divorce, and Child Custody*

As science likened women to children, so too did the legal system. Personal autonomy for women was not recognized in Victorian law and society; in a pattern typical of patriarchal power dynamics (Rubin 1975), as a young woman left her childhood home and transitioned to the domestic sphere as a wife, not only her property but also her body came under the ownership and control of her husband. For much of the nineteenth century, marriage and divorce laws codified this double standard in the legal treatment of married women. Upon marriage, the husband assumed absolute possession of all personal property his wife owned (money, stocks, household goods, and other possessions), although a husband could not will away his wife's personal "paraphernalia" such as clothing and jewelry (Combs 2004, 2005, 2006). Until 1870 a wife did not have control over her own earnings, even for income received from work undertaken separately from her husband. In the case of marriages involving land and other forms of "real" (versus personal) property, the husband was granted a "freehold estate" to such property during his wife's lifetime, at which point ownership would pass to her heir, or revert to the wife should she outlive her husband. Under equity law, such property could be settled on a woman for her separate use, but this was an expensive undertaking available only to the wealthier classes. Even a woman's body became her husband's property upon marriage, and in cases of a wife's desertion, he could file a court order for restitution of conjugal rights (Smith 1854). The concept of the wife's body as property controlled by her husband extended to cases in which women were deemed insane and committed to asylums (Showalter 1985; Oppenheim 1991; Wallis 2017).

Divorce, for the first 20 years of Victoria's reign, was nearly impossible for all but the wealthy. There were two forms of divorce: a legal separation, granted by the Ecclesiastical Courts of the Church of England, or divorce from the bonds of matrimony, through an act of Parliament. The 1857 Matrimonial Causes Act transferred juridical authority to the Court for Divorce and Matrimonial Causes and facilitated access to what was then termed a Decree of Judicial Separation, but the double standard persisted: husbands only had to prove adultery, whereas wives had to prove "aggravated adultery" (adultery plus incest, bestiality, cruelty, or desertion). The sexual double standard inherent in this distinction relied on conceptions of adultery as a violation of the husband's proprietary rights over his wife's body, and placed women in the position of having to claim victimhood in order to request separation from their spouses. However, the 1857 Act did grant separated and divorced women *feme sole* status with respect to property and legal standing, and subsequent modifications to the divorce laws in 1878, 1886, and 1895 paved the way for eventual equity for men and women under the law in the twentieth century (Horstman 1985; Shanley 1989; Hammerton 1992).

Changes to legislation surrounding Victorian marriage had significant effects on married women's ability to retain control over their own property, and bolstered early feminist campaigns for women's bodily agency and autonomy. Debates throughout the 1850s and 1860s eventually resulted in the Married Women's Property Act of 1870, which granted women such control conditionally, over property designated as "for separate use," but did not grant a married woman the same status as a *feme sole*. A modification to the law in 1874 confirmed the wife's responsibility for debts, and further modifications in 1882 finally gave married women control over property both real and personal, although since husbands could still be included in joint contracts and torts, women retained "special protections" under the law that singled them out as different than all other citizens (Stetson 1982).

Laws affecting the custody of children also fell under increasing scrutiny in the nineteenth century, particularly following the notorious case of the writer Caroline Norton, whose husband, George Norton, filed a suit for "criminal conversation" alleging adultery on the part of his wife with Lord Melbourne, then Prime Minister, in 1836. Although the jury found in favor of Lord Melbourne and Caroline Norton was deemed innocent of the charges of adultery, the law granted legal custody of the Norton's three children to their father. Throughout the 1830s Caroline Norton wrote a series of pamphlets in an effort to convince Parliament to introduce a bill redressing the inequities in the custody laws (Norton 1837, 1838, 1839). Combined with the publicity of *Norton v. Melbourne*, these pamphlets paved the way for the passage of the Custody of Infants Act (1839), which granted mothers the right to appeal for custody of children under age seven, and access to children under age 16. Norton went on to write a number of additional texts addressing the inequities in the Victorian marriage and divorce laws, and her writings were influential in the passage of the Matrimonial Causes Act in 1857 (Norton 1854, 1855). And as the laws affecting marriage, divorce, and married women's property changed, so too did the laws affecting the custody and upbringing of children: by 1873, additional legislation allowed women to petition for the right to custody over older children, and the 1886 Guardianship of Infants Act underscored the shift in focus implied in earlier legislation to emphasize the welfare of children, rather than the rights of the father, as the guideline for custody decisions.

Although the efforts to reform the Victorian marriage and divorce laws were led by women of the upper and middle classes, working-class women benefited from changes to the property laws as well as legislative changes such as the Matrimonial Causes Act of 1878, which enabled women to apply for a protection order from their local magistrate and effectively functioned as an affordable form of judicial separation. Domestic violence featured prominently in debates over the welfare of working-class married women in the 1870s: Frances Power Cobbe's 1878 exposé "Wife-Torture in England" brought attention to the exploitation and abuse of wives. Legislation in the latter part of the nineteenth century further modified these Acts by requiring husbands to pay child support in cases of desertion, and by allowing wives to leave their husbands before petitioning for a separation order on the basis of "persistent cruelty" or "wilful neglect to provide reasonable maintenance." All told, this legislation went a long way towards redressing the structural inequities in the Victorian legal treatment of wives and mothers.

### *Outside the Bonds of Marriage: Single Motherhood*

The perception and treatment of Victorian single mothers varied significantly depending on class and marital status. Widows from the upper and middle classes, if provided with monetary support in the way of a settlement or inheritance from their fathers or husbands, could maintain their social position and respectability, although the risk of financial instability remained, especially if they were not themselves expected to earn an income (Jalland 1996; Strange 2005; Heath 2009). Working-class widowed mothers had to balance the need to support and care for their children with the necessity of maintaining employment, a situation that often led to elder children, family members or neighbors providing care for younger members of the family. Following the Matrimonial Causes Act of 1878 and the infant custody legislation detailed above, if a woman wished to separate from her husband on the grounds of adultery, cruelty, or two years' wrongful desertion, she could apply for separation and maintenance for their children. In such cases, single mothers were less subject to social stigmatization than were those who themselves were charged with such breaches to the marriage contract, but it was still extremely difficult to raise children without the economic and social support systems built into the structure of Victorian marriage.

Unwed mothers were in an entirely different situation, as the very facts of pregnancy and the existence of a child were considered tantamount to declaring their disregard for the ideology of women's purity, chastity, and self-restraint. Although needless to say, there were two parties to an act of sexual intercourse resulting in the birth of a child, the woman, if unmarried, invariably bore the burden of responsibility, both legally and in the eyes of society (Levine-Clark 2004). A promise of marriage was enough to lift the cultural prescription against premarital intercourse; in cases of abandonment, the woman then had to raise the child on her own (as lawsuits for breach of promise were expensive and therefore out of reach for all but the rich) (Frost 1995; Lettmaier 2010). Privileged women were far less likely to remain single if they become pregnant outside of marriage, given the strict parental supervision they experienced and the ensuing control over their sexual and reproductive knowledge, as well as the requirement to marry. If an upper- or middle-class woman did become pregnant and were to remain unmarried, she and her family were more able to shield the existence of a child, in some cases traveling abroad for the birth and then placing the child up for adoption, in others passing off the child as the offspring of a relative after the woman's confinement.

Working-class women, who were more vulnerable to being seen as sexually available, were inevitably at risk of seduction at best, sexual assault at worst, and a pregnancy that resulted from either scenario was seen as the woman's responsibility. Whether employed as a domestic servant, or in the agricultural, industrial, or retail trades, once an unmarried woman's pregnancy was discovered, she would immediately be fired and given no references for future employment. The only recourse for working-class pregnant women was often the workhouse, which under the New Poor Law legislation (see Chapter 2) was a destination all but the most destitute strove to avoid, not only for their high infant mortality rates, but also for the perceived loss of character associated with time spent in the workhouse. Charitable organizations might step in to assist "fallen women"—the period's term for women who had borne an illegitimate child, become pregnant, or otherwise demonstrated sexual activity outside of marriage—but the associated stigma was so great that it was difficult for women to remain respectable (Anderson 1993; Sheetz-Nguyen 2012).

Once a baby was born, if a single mother without family members or other sources of support needed to work or seek employment and could not care for her infant, she might be forced to put her child up for adoption, or board the child with a neighbor paid for that purpose. The high rates of abuse and death of infants in the so-called "baby farms" of the period—unregulated residential environments in which infants were placed with wet-nurses or other caretakers while their mothers worked—provoked great concern over the welfare of poor children (Matus 1995).

By the 1870s, a parliamentary committee was charged with investigating conditions on baby farms, ultimately leading to the Infant Life Protection Act of 1872 (Arnot 1994; Homrighaus 2001). This legislation required those receiving payment for sheltering infants to register with local authorities, although it was not enforceable by law until an amendment was passed in 1897. Such legislation, combined with the various forms of protective legislation for mothers and children described in Chapter 3, eventually led to substantial improvements in the welfare and health of single mothers and their children, although it was not until the twentieth century that modern conceptions of equal parental responsibility were codified into English law.

### *Resisting the Norm: Spinsterhood and Sex Work*

Women who lived outside the norm of marriage and heterosexual domesticity occupied two extremes in the Victorian era. As noted in Chapter 2, Victorian spinsters were identified with the category of "superfluous" or "odd" women: women who whether by choice, or as a result of demographic imbalances due to emigration and other factors, remained unmarried.[1] Victorian novels from Elizabeth Gaskell's *Cranford* (1853) to Wilkie Collins's *The Woman in White* (1860) to George Gissing's *The Odd Women* (1893) depicted the spinster, maiden aunt, or unconventional unmarried middle-class woman as an asexual being whose desires were appropriately channeled into quasi-maternal activities, philanthropic work, or other forms of industrious labor. Although frequently satirized in Victorian fiction, the spinster made it possible for women to imagine and live an alternative to marriage and motherhood, and the figure of the spinster was taken up and reclaimed by many writers in the later nineteenth and early twentieth centuries as emblematic of the possibilities of a fulfilling single life (Holtby 1935; Vicinus 1985; Liggins 2016).

By contrast, Victorian sex workers (termed "prostitutes" during the period, a convention we follow here in keeping with the sociological literature of the era) were seen as overly sexual women who had succumbed to their baser instincts, whether as a result of a sexual fall or due to a supposedly "natural" tendency toward corruption and moral depravity. Such a narrative belies the reality of the majority of sex workers' lives: many pursued prostitution on a casual rather than regular basis, sometimes in the interstices of other forms of employment, sometimes as the only recourse for sustenance. Prostitution and other forms of sex work left Victorian women vulnerable to exploitation and assault, whether by clients or by the medical establishment (Walkowitz 1980, 1992). Nineteenth-century debates over the causes, effects, and amelioration of sex work led eventually to legislation intended to address concerns around the transmission of venereal disease, but also resulted in reforms led by feminist campaigners for women's rights over their own bodies, and ultimately to broader legislative changes in the twentieth century (Walkowitz 1980; Bartley 2000).

The term "prostitute" in the nineteenth century, and the broader (and vaguer) term "fallen women," encompassed much more than women who sold their bodies for sex (Flanders 2014). Contemporary writers did not necessarily distinguish between women who regularly practiced sex work as a trade, women who engaged in casual or temporary forms of prostitution, women who engaged in sexual activity out of wedlock, and women who bore illegitimate children. William Acton's *Prostitution* (1857) purported to address the health and morality of prostitutes in the era, but its assumptions regarding the causes of prostitution were founded on Victorian understandings of gender and sexuality as in need of regulation and control. In Acton's view, the demand for prostitution arose from men's "ill-regulated and uncontrolled desire," and the supply was "derived from the vice of women," resulting from a catalogue of errors: "Natural desire. Natural sinfulness. The preferment of indolent ease to labour. Vicious inclinations strengthened and ingrained by early neglect, or evil training, bad associates, and an indecent mode of life" (Acton 1857, 165). Although Acton also remarks upon the fact that prostitution might arise from "necessity, imbued by the inability to obtain a living by honest means consequent on a fall from virtue" or by "extreme poverty," his link between prostitution, vice, and the loss of virtue embodies the Victorian attitude toward sex work as the epitome of moral depravity. Notably, he also blames women for their "love of drink, love of dress, [and] love of amusement," especially those women "peculiarly exposed to temptation" as a result of their employment as actresses, milliners, shop girls, domestic servants, and factory and agricultural workers (Acton 1857, 165, 180). Acton recognized that the low wages paid to women employed in these trades were a contributing factor in leading women to "surrender their bodies to evil uses" (1857, 180), but stops short of an economic analysis that would call for changes to wages and working conditions.

The initial publication of Acton's book (1857), and his comparisons to other European nations where prostitution was legally regulated, led to the implementation of the Contagious Diseases Acts in the 1860s and the repeal campaign led by feminist reformers in subsequent decades. The repeal of the Contagious Diseases Acts in 1886 was a significant victory for the early feminist movement (although the term "feminist" itself was not in wide use at this time), and complemented the concurrent efforts for women's access to higher education and the professions as well as the first decades of the struggle for women's enfranchisement (Sanders 2015). Moreover, the repeal campaign provided women with a language and a political strategy for activism around women's sexual agency and autonomy, which were crucial elements of women's effort to control their reproductive choices as the century progressed.

### *The Skeletal Record and Sexually Transmitted Diseases*

Scholars in the fields of social history and women's history have done much to illuminate our understanding of the lived experience of Victorian sex workers (Bartley 2000; Spongberg 1997). But the addition of medical and osteological data can help deepen our understanding of the prevalence of sexually transmitted infections (often referred to as venereal diseases) for women in the nineteenth century. Sex work is often invisible or discounted in historical and social analysis, but sexually transmitted diseases, such as syphilis, were closely associated with sex work and are recorded in nineteenth-century medical texts. Such records can be used to understand the cultural implications of sexually transmitted diseases, and should also be considered when skeletal remains are examined. For the Victorian sex worker, infections related to sexual encounters may not have been well understood, yet as the nineteenth century progressed they were recognized by social activists as well as medical practitioners. Useful data can be found in the medical documentation of illness and in the developing field of vital statistics, which were being used to understand the prevalence of different diseases (Marshall 1837, Wakley 1885, Hanley 2017). In these sources we see particular attention to categorizing the developing epidemic of venereal disease, particularly in the later nineteenth century and in the decades leading up to the First World War (Royal Commission on Venereal Disease 1916). High rates of venereal disease, syphilis in particular, are also noted for the Victorian period, and structured turn-of-the-century discourses critiquing male profligacy as well as the binary depiction of the sexual depravity of prostitutes and the vulnerability of proper (married) women (Szreter 2014; Sanders 2006).

Today our knowledge of sexually transmitted diseases is well documented.[2] While HIV-AIDS is a modern health condition, others, like syphilis, have been part of the human condition for centuries. In the nineteenth century, if an individual was infected with syphilis, there was little understanding of treatment, and essentially no cure. The long-term health consequences that arise from infections like syphilis can now be well managed with antibiotics, and if infected an individual can be cured through the administering of a proper course of medication; if left untreated, however, syphilis can have serious health consequences and often lead to death.

Syphilis is a treponemal infection[3] and is transmitted through skin-to-skin contact, most often sexual contact.[4] Lesions can appear on the soft mucus membranes found in the vagina and anus, and in the mouth, but tend to last only three to six weeks at this primary stage of the disease. The secondary stage of the disease results in rashes, swollen lymph nodes and fevers, but often these two stages result in minimal to no discomfort, and may be missed. In fact, in cases of infection, "about 70 per cent of women and 55 per cent of men are largely asymptomatic and so may be unaware of their infectious carrier status, which may last for years" (McFalls and McFalls 1984, 262). It is often in this second stage of the disease that bone may begin to be impacted (Buckley and Dias 2002). If left untreated, symptoms will go away, but the underlying infection still exists in the body in what is called the latent stage, which can last for many years with no signs or symptoms, although the bone may still be reactive during this phase. The final or tertiary stage can impact different organ systems, as well as the brain and nervous systems and the skeleton, and occurs 10 to 15 years after being infected. In this phase the infection leaves additional skeletal markers; the bones hold the traces of this history.

Skeletal evidence of venereal (or secondary) syphilis and the patterns that the lesions leave behind are well established and recognizable in the clinical and skeletal anthropology literature (Steinbock 1976; Ortner and Putschar 1981; Buckley and Dias 2002). In venereal syphilis, during the secondary and latent phases of the disease the tibia (shinbones) are most often affected, bilaterally and symmetrically; the clavicle, femur, ulna, hands and feet, are also likely to reveal syphilitic markers (Buckley and Dias 2002). In the tertiary stage the frontal bone of the cranium is often the most affected (Buckley and Dias 2002). With the lack of antibiotics in the nineteenth century, the fact that there is a long dormant stage of this disease, and the indication from Victorian medical documents that syphilis was a silent epidemic, we would expect that sex workers would present skeletally with a high incidence of markers on their bodies. While a limited number of studies do exist that add to our understanding of the health consequences of Victorian sex work (Szreter 2014; Darby 2015), fewer focus directly on skeletal data to assess the impact of sexually transmitted diseases on female health and wellness in nineteenth-century England. This is a promising arena for further research in bioarchaeology and biocultural analysis.

***Contraception, Abortion, and Family Planning***

Given the dominant ideology around female sexuality during the Victorian period, it is perhaps unsurprising that methods of family planning were contingent on knowledge disseminated largely through informal networks. Although there were numerous techniques available to prevent conception in the nineteenth century, by far the most widely practiced were *coitus interruptus*, or male withdrawal before ejaculation, and abstinence (McLaren 1978; Hoggart 2003; Steinbach 2004; Szreter 2014). Abstaining from sexual intercourse was considered appropriate in a culture that valued restraint and self-control, and some Victorian couples may have timed their pregnancies by refraining from sex when they did not want to conceive a child. Condoms, sponges, diaphragms, pessaries, and other mechanical means for preventing conception were available and used by a small minority of the population; however, such methods of contraception were seen as lacking in respectability and as an interference with woman's divinely ordained (and socially constructed) role (McLaren 1978).

Women had long shared information about herbs and medicines that could be used to terminate an unplanned pregnancy, and various abortifacients in the form of patent medicines were widely advertised to bring on a woman's menstrual period (Shuttleworth 1990). Abortion itself was subject to various forms of legislation over the course of the century: although an 1803 law made it a felony to provide an abortion before fetal movements could be felt and a capital crime afterward, this gave pregnant women more authority in determining the presence of a fetus, and subsequent laws in 1828 and 1837 made abortion illegal in all cases except under certain instances and only when performed by a doctor (Steinbach 2004).

In general, it was only late in the century that forms of contraception other than abstinence and withdrawal began to be used, and they were slow to be adopted: in 1910 only one in six couples used mechanical methods of birth control, and such methods were primarily used by the middle and upper classes (Steinbach 2017). Despite extensive campaigns in the later nineteenth and early twentieth centuries, it was not until after World War I, particularly following the publication of Marie Stopes's bestselling manuals *Married Love* (1918) and *Wise Parenthood* (1919) that contraceptive practices began to be more widely used by women in England (Hoggart 2003; Debenham 2014).

## Maternal Experiences

In the Victorian period sex was seen largely as a reproductive matter, despite evidence to the contrary.[5] For Victorian couples, controlling fertility and conception was not easy, and expectations for childbearing were assumed for married women. Childbirth was defined as a woman's duty and her most rewarding purpose in life (Moscucci 1990; Marland 2004). But pregnancy, childbirth, and childrearing were often stressful and exhausting, particularly for working women, and women who already had other children (Steinbach 2004). In the case of elite women, the cultural emphasis on limited food intake, widespread corset use (in some cases, exacerbated by tight-lacing), and reduced physical activity also affected their health before, during, and after pregnancy. Multiple births over the years, coupled with nutritional stressors, hard work or lack of activity, social standards associated with the performance of proper femininity, and the shift of birth into clinical settings had a substantial impact on morbidity and mortality profiles of Victorian women when they became pregnant, gave birth, and if they survived, how they fared in the postpartum.

### *Pregnancy*

While there is little written on the direct experience of pregnancy from the perspective of the pregnant woman, medical doctors offered different types of advice. One prominent example may be seen as the nineteenth-century version of the modern tome *What To Expect When You're Expecting*, written for the middle- and upper-class woman by Dr. Pye Henry Chavasse: *Advice to a Wife on the Management of Her Own Health and on the Treatment of Some of the Complaints Incidental to Pregnancy, Labor, and Suckling, With an Introductory Chapter Especially Addressed to a Young Wife* (1842). Chavasse's manual went into multiple editions and continued to be reprinted into the twentieth century, forming part of an extensive body of advice manuals and guides for women on the management of children, on how to be a wife, and on the physical lives and health of both sexes.

Pregnancy was often a way of life for women of all classes, although working-class women typically had more children. Many Victorian women had eight or more pregnancies, although since infant mortality was high, on average only five might live until adulthood (Chavasse and Barnes 1898; Loudon 1997; Szreter and Garrett 2000). After 1860, birth rates began to decline: "between 1837 and 1851, women who married in their twenties had between 5.9 and 7.4 children, during the early 1890s women who married at the same age had only 3.3 to 5.1 children" (Steinbach 2004, 6). While fewer children were born to upper-class women, often because they had access to education and means to avoid pregnancy, their children were also more likely to survive, making the pressure to reproduce less.

While medicine worked to create a set of medically understood, clearly marked stages of pregnancy (Figure 4.1), much was still unknown about the exact processes of conception and gestation in the early Victorian period. As

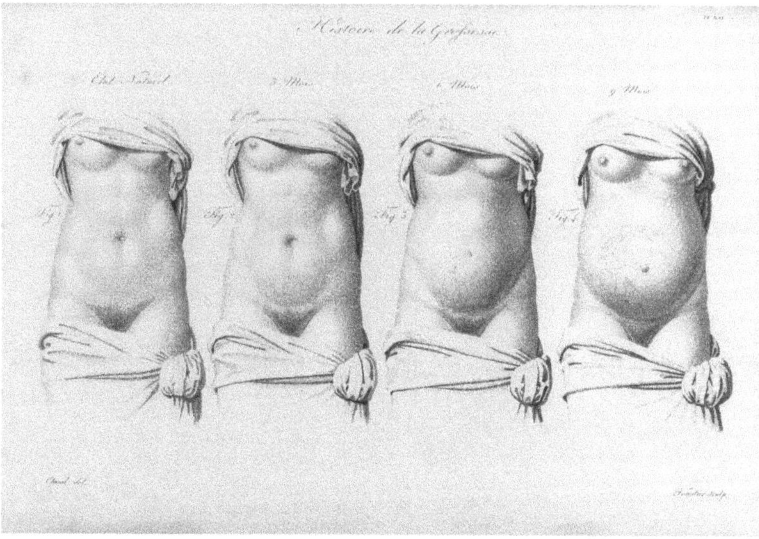

*Figure 4.1* "The Stages of Pregnancy" (Maygrier 1822, 73). Public domain.

it is today, the first month of pregnancy was often overlooked, as symptoms would not be recognized until the first menstrual period was missed. Early pregnancy, or the first trimester, was often referred to through euphemistic phrases such as "ceasing to be unwell," meaning the reduction or cessation of the monthly period (Chavasse and Barnes 1898). Other symptoms of early pregnancy included morning sickness and changes in the breasts and nipples, including shooting or throbbing pain, swelling and soreness, expression of milk, and darkening of the areolas, all of which typically occur in the first three months of pregnancy. All of these indicators were evidence of an impending pregnancy, but it was not until the expectant mother felt the "quickening," or the first movements of the developing fetus, that a pregnancy would be confirmed (Steinbach 2004). For the Victorian mother-to-be, this meant a shift in outward appearance, as the growing pregnancy became visually obvious. At this stage the traditional corset was put aside for the pregnancy corset, which allowed for less constriction and accommodated room for the growing baby (Figure 4.2).

For poor women, a pregnancy corset might also help to hide a pregnancy so that they could continue working without risk of being fired or let go; there was no legislation in place to prevent such firings until late in the twentieth century (Bach 2019).

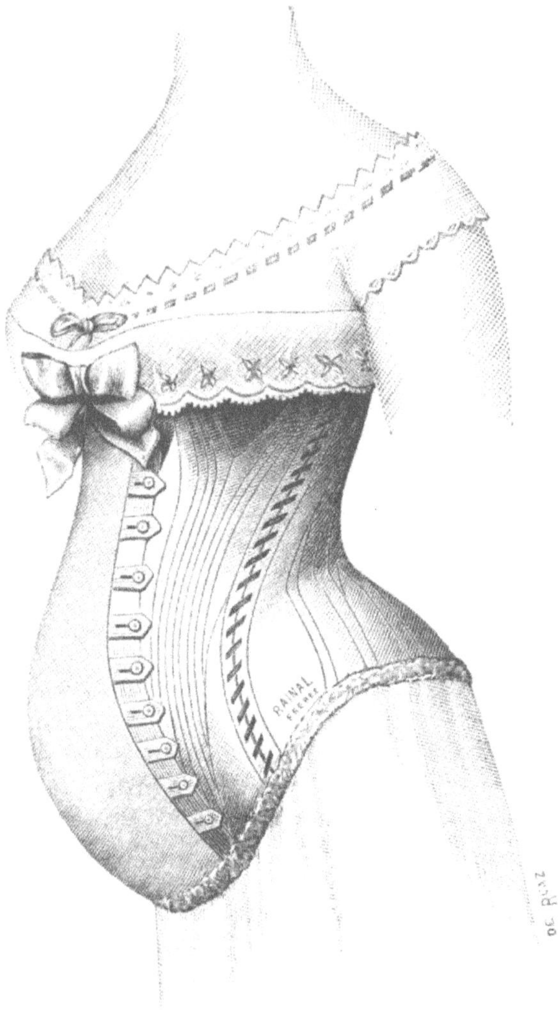

*Figure 4.2* Pregnancy corset. Credit: Wikimedia Commons, Public domain. https://commons.wikimedia.org/wiki/File:Pregnant_corset.gif

The last trimester of pregnancy presented a number of challenges for women from all classes. It was firmly believed that pregnant women in the last trimester should enter into "confinement," meaning that they would withdraw from public activity and remain at home for the duration of the pregnancy. The underpinnings of this practice are cultural as well as physiological. Confinement meant that a woman could take her corset off, remain un-corseted throughout the day, and wear less structured and less formal garments; it also meant that during the final months of pregnancy women would only to be seen by their immediate family (and domestic servants in the case of elite women). Although confinement would have been experienced differently by women of different classes—for example, both middle- and working-class women continued to care for children and undertake domestic tasks up until labor began—some of the consequences would have been shared across classes (Lewis 1984; Steinbach 2004). Not only were pregnant women confined physically to the home, they may also have become separated from existing friendship networks, emotionally and mentally confined to a distinct spatial and temporal realm that, although temporary, must have caused a sense of both eager anticipation and also loneliness and isolation. Further, for the poor the late stages of pregnancy also meant a loss of income. Childbirth as well as the early months of mothering contributed to feelings of isolation and sometimes led to morbid impacts on the parturient female body.

### *Childbirth*

Prior to the Victorian era, childbirth was most often conducted in the home and overseen by a local woman, mothers and other female relatives, and/or a midwife, making it a social and community event. This may have eased the confinement and isolation of the final trimester of pregnancy. The shift of the childbirth environment during the Victorian period from hearth and home into the evolving clinical settings, most often in the form of lying-in hospitals, and into the hands of newly minted male providers in obstetric care resulted in a dramatic increase in maternal death. The period's increase in maternal morbidity and mortality was the result of the rise in puerperal sepsis (also known as puerperal fever and childbed fever)[6], an infection transmitted through the doctors who were attending births in the lying-in hospitals (Lewis 1984; Loudon 1997). In addition, a number of studies have suggested that elite women likely suffered higher maternal death rates than did women in the general population, as they were the ones able to afford and access this new clinical care (Peller 1965; Stone 2009). Even as recently as 1932, the British Ministry of Health reported that wives in the upper and middle classes were more likely to die in childbirth than were their working-class counterparts (Chamberlain 2006).

As medicine became standardized and tied to education, and therefore transformed into a largely male endeavor, new social ideals created a manufactured sense of dependency on the medical system, which allowed for the appropriation of pregnancy and birth from the realm of women into the control of male practitioners (Ehrenreich and English 1973). Paralleling this development is the introduction in Europe of lying-in hospitals and maternity wards, which mark the first attempts to bring "parturition under professional medical care in a secular institutional setting" (Versluysen 1981,19). For the elite and those living in urban settings, clinical care in a lying-in hospital was becoming the expected way to give birth. This shift was directly influenced by the Victorian preoccupation with science, and newly developing medical systems of care for all aspects of life. Queen Victoria herself described pregnancy as "an unhappy condition" (Fulford 1964); this was a mode of relating to the experience of pregnancy and birth that underscored cultural perceptions of labor and childbirth as traumatic, in keeping with the biblical prescription that painful labors were a form of punishment for Eve's original sin. Victoria used chloroform in the births of two of her children (Leopold in 1853 and Beatrice in 1857), and subsequently the use of anesthetics in childbirth became more common, particularly among the upper classes (Gibbs 1987).

Lying-in hospitals were the foundational clinical setting for childbirth. Here large dormitory spaces were constructed for women to "lie-in" as they went through labor and childbirth (Figure 4.3). While all appearances suggested a controlled and monitored space, the lying-in hospital was far from sterile. Doctors would attend one woman after another, often coming in from an autopsy or other surgery without washing their hands (Chamberlain 2006). At the start of the Victorian period there was no sense of germ theory (that came in 1881 with Louis Pasteur's work), so hand-washing between patients was not a common practice. While others had recognized the impact of washing hands on the reduction of infectious disease transmission, changes in the care of pregnant women, decreasing the infection rates, did not gain traction until the early 1930s (Chamberlain 2006). For Victorian women, especially from the middle and upper classes, this meant that the risk for maternal death as a result of childbirth was high, and this degree of risk generated a new focus for medical science to understand why. Unfortunately, the explanations for increases in maternal deaths focused on pathologizing pregnancy and the birth process, instead of looking to the larger systemic issues of medical care as contributing to maternal death.

### *Maternal Mortality: Medicine and Childbed Death*

The dramatic and unprecedented increase in the incidence of childbed death stemming directly from clinical care was emblematic of the Victorian era. Puerperal sepsis and pyrexia, which takes hold three to ten days after birth, are both the result of unsanitary conditions that lead to bacterial infections of the birth canal (Loudon 1992; Chamberlain 2006). These infections were

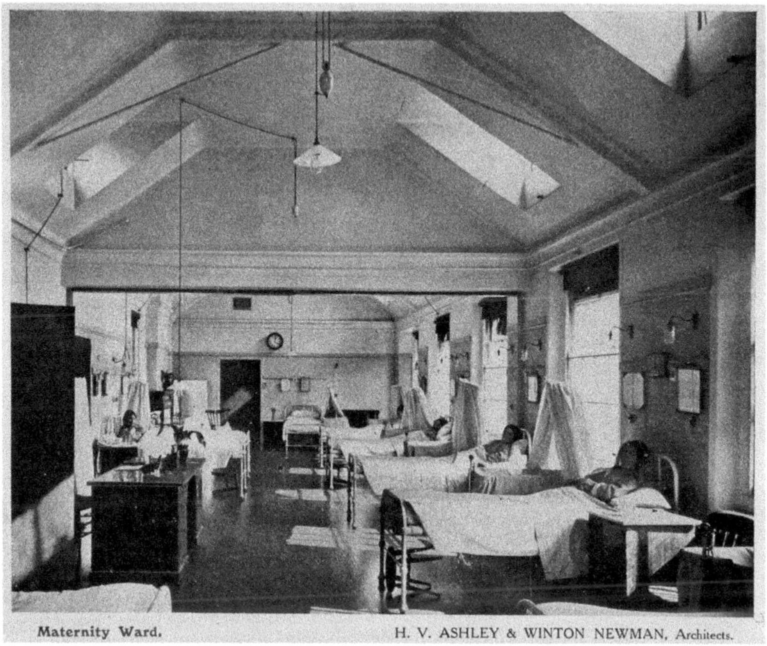


*Figure 4.3* Royal Free Hospital, London: the interior of the maternity ward, 1913. Credit: Wellcome Collection. https://wellcomecollection.org/works/dr799ure

the most common cause of maternal death in this period, impacting between 30 and 50 percent of all parturient females. "between 1847 and 1903, 93,342 deaths from puerperal fevers were recorded in England and Wales, and this is almost certainly an underestimate of the true total" (Figure 4.4) (Loudon 1992, 49). Without antibiotics for women who contracted bacterial infections as a result of giving birth in lying-in hospitals as well as with doctors in their homes, death was almost inevitable. While the introduction of bacteria leading to infection was almost always the result of the clinical environment and the lack of hygienic practices by doctors, those that cast the blame on them were quickly silenced. For example, the physician Ignaz Semmelweis determined that medical students at the Vienna General Hospital were conveying infection to women in labor as a result of failing to wash their hands after postmortem dissections, and in 1847 he proved that washing with carbolic soap substantially decreased the rate of puerperal fever. Nonetheless, he was roundly criticized by fellow obstetricians (Chamberlain 2006).

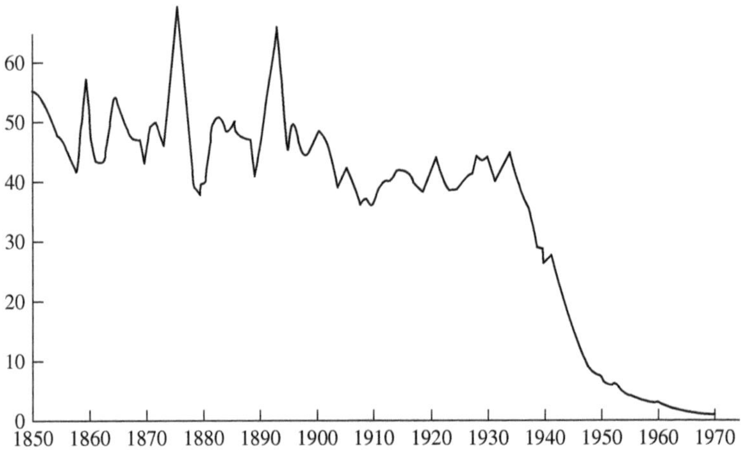


*Figure 4.4* "Annual death rate per 1,000 total births from maternal mortality in England and Wales (1850–1970) (Registrar General Reports)" (from Chamberlain 2006, 560).

In addition to sepsis, the Victorian era saw other causes of death resulting from childbirth that are recognized today, including hemorrhage, placenta praevia[7], abruption of the placenta[8], and preeclampsia[9] (also known as toxemia), all of which were not understood until the mid-twentieth century, and all of which vex parturient women today as well (in much smaller numbers to be sure). Other issues relating to obstructed labors amplified the degree of risk, as surgery was often needed, but operations such as the caesarean section were considered only in extreme cases since they were likely to result in the death of mother or baby, if not both (Moscucci 1990; Nielsen 1995).

Prior to the nineteenth century, cesarean section was used only in rare and desperate cases (Nielsen 1995). In the eighteenth century, mortality associated with cesarean section was reported to be 80 to 90 percent, only falling 4 to 10 percent by the first part of the twentieth century (Nielsen 1995). In comparison, in the later part of the twentieth century, even with improvements in medical care, mortality rates as a result of cesarean section are still estimated to be 10 to 20 times higher than the rate of mortality for women who give birth vaginally (Nielsen 1995). Despite innovations in the type of incision and the sutures used to avoid uterine rupture in subsequent pregnancies, it was not until the introduction of antibiotics in the twentieth century that maternal mortality resulting from complications from cesarean sections decreased significantly.

Given these medical and environmental factors, we can begin to understand how the shift to clinical birth settings set the stage for higher risk of death in childbed in the Victorian period; but cultural practices also had a role in these deaths in childbed. The incidence of complications due to obstructed labor was likely influenced by long-term corset use and the use of corsets to disguise pregnancy. Exacerbated by the nutritional deficiencies discussed in Chapter 3, these cultural practices resulted in changes to the skeletal structure that had serious implications for maternal as well as infant mortality.

While maternal infection rates (particularly sepsis) were dramatically increased by the use of lying-in hospitals and unsanitary conditions, the addition of obstructed labors as the result of the flattened pelvis created further complications and fueled the skyrocketing maternal mortality rates of the Victorian era (Loudon 1992, 1997; Stone 2009, 2016). Many scholars have identified the flattened pelvis as a primary risk indicator for obstructed labor (Caldwell and Moloy 1938; Wells et al. 2012), and as noted in Chapter 3, the flattening of the pelvis could be brought on by diseases such as rickets. While rickets alone could not account for the high incidence of obstructed labors as a result of a contracted pelvis in the Victorian period, the combination of rickets, flattened pelvic architecture, and giving birth in the clinical setting contributed to the high rates of maternal death at this time (Loudon 1997; Stone 2009, 2012, 2016).

Why was labor and birth seemingly so different for Victorian women than for women today? As evidenced in the literature that documents rising maternal mortality rates over the course of the nineteenth century, the compromised pelvis did lead to increased difficulties in childbirth in the Victorian era. Problems that resulted from a rachitic pelvis, exacerbated by corset use, can be traced to nutritional deficiencies and environmental conditions as well as ideologies associated with proper femininity. However, interpretations of high rates of maternal mortality for white women were used to advance biologically deterministic typological ideas of racial differences, making death in childbed a flaw of the female body and not the result of specific cultural practices. While the shift in the birthing experience from the home to the clinical environment brought with it a litany of potential risks for Victorian women, many conformed to the new standards of care and sought out hospitals and clinics in which to give birth. From infections to cesarean delivery and ultimately death, childbirth came to be considered a risky endeavor, influencing generations of women's choices and perceptions of labor and birth. In turn, the medicalization of birth likely put the nineteenth-century mother at higher risk for complications associated with the stresses of parturition and maternity than had been seen in previous populations (Stone 2016).

The culture of medicine that developed through socially imposed factors significantly affected the health and lifestyle of women across classes in nineteenth-century England. Social and moral ideals, combined with the medical need for uniform practices in the training of physicians and specifically with respect to obstetrics, resulted in the construction of standards used to make clinical measurements of pelvic shape and size uniform in an effort to evaluate and mitigate the maternal risk of obstructed labor. These standards, which are still in place today, use culturally determined definitions of human biology that assume a static and unchanging picture of the human body. Moreover, they are based on early evolutionary studies and racial typologies and disregard the variable nature of human biology and cultural changes through time. It is critical that modern studies begin to examine the links between changes in social identity, health, and the medical management of parturition, not only as they have had a lasting effect on the way in which women's bodies are assessed, but as a means to understand why pregnancy and particularly birth have been problematized by history and not necessarily by the parturient body.

## *Babies, Breastfeeding, and a Lifetime of Motherhood*

> A wife is now about to assume an additional and higher title than that of Wife, namely, that of Mother.
>
> (Chavasse and Barnes 1898, 242)

Not much is written about the experiences of mothering from the perspective of Victorian mothers themselves. Exceptions may be found in literary texts, especially in the vein of sentimental fiction, which was considered the particular province of women writers; and occasionally, women's diaries and letters can offer a glimpse into the lived experience of motherhood in the Victorian period (Davies 1915). Fictional representations of motherhood in the Victorian period reproduced the image of the ideal mother as fulfilling cultural expectations of respectability, femininity, stability, and domestic virtue (McKnight 1997). The advice offered to women in the form of manuals addressing reproductive health was deeply intertwined with social assumptions about the knowledge that women (specifically, white middle- and upper-class women) lacked as they became pregnant, labored, birthed, and suckled (breastfed their infants). Working-class women, by contrast, were assumed to already have the necessary knowledge surrounding reproduction and birth, but these assumptions were also class-bound and shaped by stereotypes of working-class sexuality and family life.

Breastfeeding was seen as an important part of the transition into motherhood, but it also added a socially scripted set of rules that added to the sense of isolation new mothers felt. For poor women already suffering from nutritional deprivation and exhaustion, breastfeeding may have felt like an additional burden on the body in addition to depleting the resources of the family. Breastfeeding was thought to be a method of controlling fertility; some women nursed their babies for longer periods of time in order to space pregnancies or limit the likelihood of conception, but many working women had no choice but to wean their infants in order to return to work (Steinbach 2004). For the middle and upper classes, suckling was carried out at home, and hidden from public view; some elite women hired wet-nurses to suckle their children (Lewis 1986, cited in Steinbach 2004). Many doctors presumed that a new mother would be able to stay at home for a number of months after the birth in order to breastfeed according to a strict schedule: "For the first month the child should be suckled every hour and a half, for the second month every two hours, gradually lengthening the distance of time between as the child becomes older, till at length he has it about every four hours" (Chavasse 1844, 74). The recommendations were to wean a child between the ages of six months "if the mother be weak," and twelve months "if the child be weak or labouring under any disease," but in general, the conclusion was that "nine months is the most proper time" for weaning (Chavasse 1844, 88). In determining a schedule for breastfeeding and recommended times for weaning, the medical rationale for these recommendations was not articulated; nevertheless, such guidelines set the stage for the recommendations for breastfeeding and weaning that are still in place today.

Like many of his era, Chavasse also offered advice meant to support the young mother as she shifted into her new role. His popular text *Advice to a Mother in the Management of her Offspring* (originally published in 1834, with revised editions dating into the 1860s), reveals how Victorian ideologies of motherhood intertwines with medical advice regarding the care of children and the role of the mother in the family. As the century progressed, advice manuals and conduct guides proliferated, although their recommendations often paralleled the literature of the era, in which mothers were idealized as angelic providers and exhorted to attend carefully to the momentous responsibilities associated with their role in the family and in society (Ellis 1843). Alternatively, mothers in Victorian fiction are absent altogether, and therefore culpable by default as their children grow up without guidance. Many of these missing mothers in Victorian fiction themselves died as a result of complications from childbirth, testifying to the powerful narratives surrounding the idealization of motherhood and the tragedy and risks associated with pregnancy and birth.

These representations, bridging the medical literature and the fiction and advice manuals of the era, leave us with a complicated understanding of

Victorian discourses of mothering across classes. The increase in economic stability for the middle and upper classes, and societal expectations that women who could do so would hire help with domestic tasks in the form of nannies, nurses, and tutors, meant that some mothers might not have a substantial role in the upbringing of their children. Other women felt their lives subsumed in the experience of maternity, especially given the high birth rate in the first half of the century and the lack of access to contraceptive knowledge across classes. Many mothers bore multiple children, and among those who lived into childhood and adolescence, daughters were trained to take up the role perceived as their destiny, as wives and mothers (Ellis 1842). Mothers therefore played a vital role not only within the family, but also in Victorian society as a whole.

While there is much research that focuses on childhood and children's experiences in the nineteenth century, fewer scholars focus on the lived experience of mothering children in the Victorian era. Exceptions include a number of useful sources on working-class women, among them Ellen Ross's work on poor mothers in late nineteenth-century London (Ross 1993), and the primary accounts included in Margaret Llewelyn Davies's *Maternity: Letters from Working Women* (1915) and conveyed through oral history (Roberts 1984). These sources offer a glimpse into the lived experience of Victorian motherhood for working women; further research would help to illuminate the experience of mothering across classes and create a fuller picture of motherhood over the course of the nineteenth century.

## To Sum Up

- The Victorian model of marriage and the construction of the family meant that women struggled within the legal and social constraints of the period—whether as married women, as single women, or as women sexually active outside of marriage.
- This is a time period of women's highest reproductive capacity (late teens to 40s/50s); the reproductive body and expectations regarding motherhood were of concern throughout the era, as were alternative modes of addressing expectations for reproduction and birth (abortion and contraception).
- Women were dying in childbirth at dramatic rates in Victorian England, and this is when the standards were being set for how we conceive of childbirth (in keeping with ideological conceptions of motherhood).
- Victorian experiences of motherhood are rarely considered through direct accounts; instead we must make inferences from medical and legal texts, advice manuals, and fictional narratives.

## Questions to Consider

- Why is there little written on conception and pregnancy in the Victorian era?
- What experiences of pregnancy and birth were shared across classes, and how did these experiences differ?

## Notes

1 Indeed, Victorian spinsters were encouraged to emigrate to the colonies in order to redress this perceived imbalance and discourage interracial marriage (Krandis 1999).

2 There are many online resources with detailed information about sexually transmitted diseases and treatments. For example: https://www.cdc.gov/std/syphilis/stdfact-syphilis.htm

3 Syphilis is one of three forms of treponemal diseases (syphilis, yaws, bejel) caused by a spirochete bacterium. For more information and for skeletal discriminators, see Rothschild and Rothschild (1995).

4 Syphilis can also be transmitted from mother to unborn child through the placental barrier. In cases where a pregnant woman has syphilis it can result in low birth weight of the child, premature birth, and stillbirth; children born with congenital syphilis are likely to develop serious health issues. https://www.cdc.gov/std/syphilis/stdfact-syphilis.htm

5 In addition to non-reproductive sexual acts between married couples, there is also evidence of same-sex relationships in which sexual practices were not named, but assumed (Cook 2003; Vicinus 2004; Marcus 2007; Upchurch 2009).

6 *Puerperal sepsis* is clinically an illness that results from an infection of the uterus during or after delivery. It is rarely seen today.

7 *Placenta praevia* "is a condition where the placenta lies low in the uterus and partially or completely covers the cervix. The placenta may separate from the uterine wall as the cervix begins to dilate (open) during labor," resulting in the placenta blocking the path of the neonate. This condition requires a cesarean section. Today this impacts about 1 in 200 women. https://americanpregnancy.org/pregnancy-complications/placenta-previa/

8 *Abruption of the placenta* "is the separation of the placenta from the uterine lining. This condition usually occurs in the third trimester but can occur any time after the 20th week of pregnancy. Only about 1% of all pregnant women will experience placental abruption, and most can be successfully treated depending on what type of separation occurs." https://americanpregnancy.org/pregnancy-complications/placental-abruption/

9 *Preeclampsia/toxemia* "is a condition that occurs only during pregnancy. Some symptoms of preeclampsia may include high blood pressure and protein in the urine, occurring after week 20 of pregnancy. Preeclampsia is often precluded by gestational hypertension. While high blood pressure during pregnancy does not necessarily indicate preeclampsia, it may be a sign of another problem. Preeclampsia affects at least 5–8% of pregnancies." https://americanpregnancy.org/pregnancy-complications/preeclampsia/

## References

### Primary Sources

Acton, William. 1857. *Prostitution, Considered in Its Moral, Social, and Sanitary Aspects, in London and Other Large Cities and Garrison Towns, with Proposals for the Control and Prevention of Its Attendant Evils*. Revised edition. London: John Churchill and Sons, 1870.

Chavasse, Pye Henry. 1844. *Advice to Wives on the Management of Themselves: During the Periods of Pregnancy, Labour, and Suckling*. New York: D. Appleton and Co.

Chavasse, Pye Henry. 1860. *Advice to a Mother on the Management of Her Offspring*. 5th ed. London: John Churchill.

Chavasse, Pye Henry, and F. Barnes. 1898. *Chavasse's Advice to a Wife on the Management of Her Own Health and on the Treatment of Some of the Complaints Incidental to Pregnancy, Labor, and Suckling*. 14th ed. New York: G. Routledge & Sons, Limited.

Cobbe, Frances Power. 1878. "Wife Torture in England." *The Contemporary Review* 32 (April): 55–87. Reprinted in *Criminals, Idiots, Women, and Minors: Victorian Writing By Women on Women*, edited by Susan Hamilton, 132–169. Peterborough, ON: Broadview Press, 1995.

Collins, Wilkie. 1860. *The Woman in White*. Edited with an introduction by Matthew Sweet. London/New York: Penguin Classics, 1999.

Davies, Margaret Llewelyn, ed. 1915. *Maternity: Letters from Working Women*. London: Virago Press, 1978.

Ellis, Sarah Stickney. 1842. *The Daughters of England, Their Position in Society, Character and Responsibilities*. London: Fisher, Son, and Co.

Ellis, Sarah Stickney. 1843. *The Mothers of England, Their Influence and Responsibility*. London: Fisher, Son, and Co.

Gaskell, Elizabeth. 1853. *Cranford*. Edited with an introduction by Patricia Ingham. London/New York: Penguin Classics, 2005.

Gissing, George. 1893. *The Odd Women*. Edited by Arlene Young. Peterborough, ON: Broadview Press, 1998.

Hamilton, Cicely. 1909. *Marriage as a Trade*. New York: Moffat, Yard and Company.

Marshall, John. 1837. Royal College of Surgeons of England. *Statistics of the British Empire. Mortality of the Metropolis: A Statistical View of the Number of Persons Reported to Have Died, of Each of More Than 100 Kinds of Disease, and Casualties, Within the Bills of Mortality, in Each of the Two Hundred and Four Years, 1629–1831*. London: J. Haddon.

Norton, Caroline. 1837. *Observations on the Natural Claim of a Mother to the Custody of Her Children as Affected by the Common Law Right of the Father*. London: James Ridgway and Sons.

Norton, Caroline. 1838. *The Separation of Mother and Child by the Law of "Custody of Infants," Considered*. London: Roake and Varty.

Norton, Caroline. 1839. *A Plain Letter to the Lord Chancellor on the Infant Custody Bill*. London: James Ridgway.

Norton, Caroline. 1854. *English Laws for Women in the Nineteenth Century.* Reprinted with an introduction by Joan Huddleston. Chicago, IL: Academy Chicago Publishers, 1982.

Norton, Caroline. 1855. *A Letter to the Queen on Lord Chancellor Cranworth's Marriage and Divorce Bill.* 3rd ed. London: Longman, Brown, Green, and Longmans.

Patmore, Coventry. 1854–1862. *The Angel in the House*. London: Cassell and Co, 1887.

Ruskin, John. 1865. *Sesame and Lilies*. Edited with an introduction by Deborah Epstein Nord. New Haven, CT: Yale University Press, 2002.

Smith, Barbara Leigh [later Bodichon]. 1854. 2nd ed. revised with additions, 1856. *A Brief Summary, in Plain Language, of the Most Important Laws Concerning Women; Together with a Few Observations Thereon.* London: John Chapman.

Stopes, Marie. 1918. *Married Love: A New Contribution to the Solution of Sex Difficulties*. Oxford: Oxford World's Classics, 2004.

Stopes, Marie. 1918. *Wise Parenthood: A Sequel to "Married Love."* 5th ed. London: A. C. Fifield, 1919.

Wakley, J. G., ed. 1885. "The Contagious Disease Acts." *The Lancet: A Journal of British and Foreign Medicine, Physiology, Surgery, Chemistry, Public Health, Criticism, and News* 126 (October): 674–676.

## *Secondary Sources*

Anderson, Amanda. 1993. *Tainted Souls and Painted Faces: The Rhetoric of Fallenness in Victorian Culture*. Ithaca, NY: Cornell University Press.

Arnot, Margaret L. 1994. "Infant Death, Child Care and the State: The Baby-Farming Scandal and the First Infant Life Protection Legislation of 1872." *Continuity and Change* 9 (2): 271–311.

Bartley, Paula. 2000. *Prostitution: Prevention and Reform in England, 1860–1914*. London/New York: Routledge.

Buckley, Haile R., and George J. Dias. 2002. "The Distribution of Skeletal Lesions in Treponemal Disease: Is the Lymphatic System Responsible?" *International Journal of Osteoarchaeology* 12 (3): 178–188.

Caldwell, W. E., and H. C. Moloy. 1938. "Anatomical Variations in the Female Pelvis: Their Classification and Obstetrical Significance." *Proceedings of the Royal Society of Medicine* 32 (1): 1–30.

Chamberlain, G. 2006. "British Maternal Mortality in the 19$^{th}$ and Early 20$^{th}$ Centuries." *Journal of the Royal Society of Medicine* 99 (11): 559–563.

Combs, Mary Beth. 2004. "The Price of Independence: How the 1870 Married Women's Property Act Altered the Investment Risks Faced by Lower Middle Class British Women." *Journal of Economics* 30 (2): 1–26.

Combs, Mary Beth. 2005. "'A Measure of Legal Independence': The 1870 Married Women's Property Act and the Portfolio Allocations of British Wives." *The Journal of Economic History* 65 (4): 1028–1057.

Combs, Mary Beth. 2006. "*Cui Bono?* The 1870 British Married Women's Property Act, Bargaining Power, and the Distribution of Resources with Marriage." *Feminist Economics* 12 (1–2): 51–83.

Cook, Matt. 2003. *London and the Culture of Homosexuality, 1885–1914*. Cambridge/New York: Cambridge University Press.

Darby, Robert. 2015. "Syphilis 1855 and HIV-AIDS 2007: Historical Reflections on the Tendency to Blame Human Anatomy for the Action of Micro-organisms." *Global Public Health* 10 (5–6): 573–588.

Debenham, Clare. 2014. *Birth Control and the Rights of Women: Post Suffrage Feminism in the Early Twentieth Century*. London/New York: I. B. Tauris.

Ehrenreich, Barbara, and Deirdre English. 1973. *Witches, Midwives and Nurses: A History of Women Healers*. Old Westbury, NY: Feminist Press.

Frost, Ginger Suzanne. 1995. *Promises Broken: Courtship, Class, and Gender in Victorian England*. Charlottesville, VA: University Press of Virginia.

Fulford, Roger. 1964. *Dearest Child: Letters Between Queen Victoria and the Princess Royal, 1858–1861*. London: Evans Bros.

Gibbs, Patricia. 1987. "Lessons from Literature: Pregnancy and Childbirth." *Perspectives in Biology and Medicine* 31 (1): 94–105.

Hammerton, A. James. 1992. *Cruelty and Companionship: Conflict in Nineteenth-Century Married Life*. London/New York: Routledge.

Hanley, Anne R. 2017. *Medicine, Knowledge and Venereal Diseases in England, 1886–1916*. Cham: Springer International Publishing; Imprint: Palgrave Macmillan.

Heath, Kay. 2009. *Aging by the Book: The Emergence of Midlife in Victorian Britain*. Albany, NY: State University of New York Press.

Hochschild, Arlie, and Anne Machung. 1989. *The Second Shift: Working Families and the Revolution at Home*. New York: Viking.

Hoggart, Lesley. 2003. *Feminist Campaigns for Birth Control and Abortion Rights in Britain*. Studies in British History 69. Lewiston, NY: The Edwin Mellen Press.

Holcombe, Lee. 1983. *Wives and Property: Reform of the Married Women's Property Law in Nineteenth-Century England*. Toronto, ON/Buffalo, NY: University of Toronto Press.

Holtby, Winifred. 1935. *Women and a Changing Civilization*. Cassandra Editions. Chicago, IL: Academy Press, 1978.

Homrighaus, Ruth Ellen. 2001. "Wolves in Women's Clothing: Baby-Farming and the *British Medical Journal*, 1860–1872." *Journal of Family History* 26 (3): 350–372.

Horstman, Allen. 1985. *Victorian Divorce*. New York: St. Martin's Press.

Jalland, Pat. 1996. *Death in the Victorian Family*. Oxford: Oxford University Press.

Krandis, Rita S. 1999. *The Victorian Spinster and Colonial Emigration: Contested Subjects*. New York: St. Martin's Press.

Lettmaier, Saskia. 2010. *Broken Engagements: The Action for Breach of Promise of Marriage and the Feminine Ideal, 1800–1940*. Oxford: Oxford University Press.

Lewis, Jane. 1984. *Women in England 1870–1950: Sexual Divisions and Social Change*. Sussex: Wheatsheaf Press; Bloomington, IN: Indiana University Press.

Levine-Clark, Marjorie. 2004. *Beyond the Reproductive Body: The Politics of Women's Health and Work in Early Victorian England*. Columbus, OH: The Ohio State University Press.

Lewis, Judith S. 1986. *In the Family Way: Childbearing in the British Aristocracy, 1760–1860*. New Brunswick, NJ: Rutgers University Press.

Liggins, Emma. 2016. *Odd Women? Spinsters, Lesbians and Widows in British Women's Fiction, 1850s–1930s*. Manchester: Manchester University Press.

Loudon, Irvine. 1992. *Death in Childbirth: An International Study of Maternal Care and Maternal Mortality 1800–1950*. New York: Clarendon/Oxford University Press.

Loudon, Irvine. 1997. "Childbirth." In *Western Medicine*, edited by Irvine Loudon, 206–220. Oxford/New York: Oxford University Press.

Marcus, Sharon. 2007. *Between Women: Friendship, Desire, and Marriage in Victorian England*. Princeton, NJ: Princeton University Press.

Marland, Hilary. 2004. *Dangerous Motherhood: Insanity and Childbirth in Victorian Britain*. Basingstoke/New York: Palgrave Macmillan.

Matus, Jill L. 1995. *Unstable Bodies: Victorian Representations of Sexuality and Maternity*. Manchester and New York: Manchester University Press.

Maygrier, Jacques-Pierre. 1822. *Nouveaux élémens de la science et de l'art des accouchemens*, 73. Ouvrage illustré de 80 planches gravées en taille-douce par Forestier et François-Louis Couché fils (1782–1849), d'après Anotine Chazal. Paris: Béchet.

McFalls, Joseph A., and Marguerite Harvey McFalls. 1984. *Disease and Fertility*. New York: Academic Press.

McKnight, Natalie J. 1997. *Suffering Mothers in Mid-Victorian Novels*. New York: St. Martin's Press.

McLaren, Angus. 1978. *Birth Control in Nineteenth-Century England*. New York: Holmes and Meier.

Mitchell, Sally. 1996. *Daily Life in Victorian England*. Westport, CT/London: Greenwood Press.

Moscucci, Ornella. 1990. *The Science of Woman: Gynaecology and Gender in England, 1800–1929*. Cambridge: Cambridge University Press.

Nielsen, T. F. 1995. "Cesarean Section." In *Reproductive Health Care for Women and Babies*, edited by B. P. Sachs, R. Beard, E. Papiernlk, and C. Russell, 279–289. Oxford: Oxford University Press.

Oppenheim, Janet. 1991. *"Shattered Nerves": Doctors, Patients, and Depression in Victorian England*. New York: Oxford University Press.

Ortner, D. J., and G. J. Putschar. 1981. *Identification of Pathological Conditions in Human Skeletal Remains*. Washington, DC: Smithsonian Institution Press.

Peller, Sigismund. 1965. "Births and Deaths Among Europe's Ruling Families Since 1500." In *Population in History: Essays in Historical Demography*, edited by D. V. Glass and D. E. C. Eversley, 87–100. New York: Routledge.

Perkin, Joan. 1989. *Women and Marriage in Nineteenth-Century England*. London: Routledge.

Phegley, Jennifer. 2012. *Courtship and Marriage in Victorian England.* Santa Barbara, CA: Praeger.

Roberts, Elizabeth. 1984. *A Woman's Place: An Oral History of Working-Class Women, 1890–1940*. Oxford: Basil Blackwell.

Ross, Ellen. 1993. *Love and Toil: Motherhood in Outcast London 1870–1918*. New York/Oxford: Oxford University Press.

Rothschild, Bruce M., and Christine Rothschild. 1995. "Treponemal Disease Revisited: Skeletal Discriminators for Yaws, Bejel, and Venereal Syphilis." *Clinical Infectious Diseases* 20 (5) (May): 1402–1408.

Royal Commission on Venereal Diseases Final Report. 1916. "Royal Commission on Venereal Disease: Final Report of the Commissioners." *The Lancet* 187 (4828) (March): 575–576.

Rubin, Gayle. 1975. "The Traffic in Women: Notes on the Political Economy of Sex." In *Toward and Anthropology of Women*, edited by Rayna Reiter, 157–210. New York/London: Monthly Review Press.

Sanders, Lise Shapiro. 2006. *Consuming Fantasies: Labor, Leisure, and the London Shopgirl, 1880–1920*. Columbus, OH: The Ohio State University Press.

Sanders, Lise Shapiro. 2015. "'Equal Laws Based Upon an Equal Standard': The Garrett Sisters, the Contagious Diseases Acts, and the Sexual Politics of Victorian and Edwardian Feminism Revisited." *Women's History Review* 24 (3): 389–409.

Shanley, Mary Lyndon. 1989. *Feminism, Marriage and the Law in Victorian England, 1850–1895*. Princeton, NJ: Princeton University Press.

Sheetz-Nguyen, Jessica. 2012. *Victorian Women, Unwed Mothers and the London Foundling Hospital*. London: Continuum.

Showalter, Elaine. 1985. *The Female Malady: Women, Madness, and English Culture, 1830–1980*. New York: Penguin.

Shuttleworth, Sally. 1990. "Female Circulation: Medical Discourse and Popular Advertising in the Mid-Victorian Era." In *Body/Politics: Women and the Discourses of Science*, edited by Mary Jacobus, Evelyn Fox Keller, and Sally Shuttleworth, 47–68. New York: Routledge.

Spongberg, Mary. 1997. *Feminizing Venereal Disease: The Body of the Prostitute in Nineteenth-Century Medical Discourse*. New York: New York University Press.

Steinbach, Susie. 2004. *Women in England 1760–1914: A Social History*. New York: Palgrave Macmillan.

Steinbach, Susie L. 2017. *Understanding the Victorians: Politics, Culture and Society in Nineteenth-Century Britain*. 2nd ed. London/New York: Routledge.

Steinbock, R. 1976. *Paleopathological Diagnosis and Interpretation: Bone Diseases in Ancient Human Populations*. Springfield, IL: Charles C. Thomas.

Stetson, Dorothy. 1982. *A Woman's Issue: The Politics of Family Law Reform in England*. Westport, CT: Greenwood Press.

Stone, Pamela K. 2009. "A History of Western Medicine, Labor, and Birth." In *Childbirth Across Cultures: Ideas and Practices of Pregnancy, Birth, and the Postpartum*, edited by Helaine Selin and Pamela K. Stone, 41–53. Dordrecht: Springer.

Stone, Pamela K. 2012. "Binding Women: Ethnology, Skeletal Deformations, and Violence Against Women." *International Journal of Paleopathology* 2 (2–3): 53–60.

Stone, Pamela K. 2016. "Biocultural Perspectives on Maternal Mortality and Obstetrical Death from the Past to the Present." *American Journal of Physical Anthropology* 159: 150–171.

Strange, Julie-Marie. 2005. *Death, Grief and Poverty in Britain, 1870–1914.* Cambridge: Cambridge University Press.

Szreter, Simon. 2014. "The Prevalence of Syphilis in England and Wales on the Eve of the Great War: Re-visiting the Estimates of the Royal Commission on Venereal Diseases 1913–1916." *Social History of Medicine* 27 (3): 508–529.

Szreter, Simon, and Eilidh Garrett. 2000. "Reproduction, Compositional Demography, and Economic Growth: Family Planning in England Long Before the Fertility Decline." *Population and Development Review* 26 (1): 45–80.

Upchurch, Charles. 2009. *Before Wilde: Sex Between Men in Britain's Age of Reform*. Berkeley, CA: University of California Press, 2009.

Versluysen, M. C. 1981. "Midwives, Medical Men and 'Poor Women Labouring of Child': Lying-in Hospitals in Eighteenth-Century London." In *Women, Health and Reproduction*, edited by Helen Roberts, 18–49. London: Routledge and Kegan Paul.

Vicinus, Martha. 1985. *Independent Women: Work and Community for Single Women 1850–1920*. Chicago, IL: University of Chicago Press.

Vicinus, Martha. 2004. *Intimate Friends: Women Who Loved Women, 1778–1928.* Chicago, IL: University of Chicago Press.

Vickery, Amanda. 1993. "Golden Age to Separate Spheres: A Review of the Categories and Chronology of English Women's History." *Historical Journal* 36 (2): 383–414.

Walkowitz, Judith. 1980. *Prostitution and Victorian Society: Women, Class, and the State*. Cambridge: Cambridge University Press.

Walkowitz, Judith. 1992. *City of Dreadful Delight: Narratives of Sexual Danger in Late-Victorian London*. Chicago, IL: University of Chicago Press.

Wallis, Jennifer. 2017. *Investigating the Body in the Victorian Asylum: Doctors, Patients, and Practices*. Houndsmills, Basingstoke, Hampshire: Palgrave Macmillan.

Wells, J. C., J. M. DeSilva, and J. T. Stock. 2012. "The Obstetric Dilemma: An Ancient Game of Russian Roulette, or a Variable Dilemma Sensitive to Ecology?" *American Journal of Physical Anthropology* 149 (Supplement 55): 40–71.

### *Online Resources*

Bach, Emily. 2019. "Victorian Image of Pregnancy Through Corsetry." Maryland Historical Society. http://blog.mdhs.org/costumes/victorian-image-of-pregnancy-through-corsetry. Accessed 20 September 2019.

Flanders, Judith. 2014. "Prostitution." Discovering Literature: Romantics & Victorians, The British Library. https://www.bl.uk/romantics-and-victorians/articles/prostitution. Accessed 18 June 2019.

# 5 Matriarchs, Menopause, and Death

## Introduction

Life after reproduction is often neglected when we discuss the past, particularly when we focus on women's lives. Cross-culturally there are many different ways in which the elder members of communities are considered, revered, and even supported. However, the Victorian period seems to be the originator of how the Western world today approaches aging, often resulting in the elderly being removed from society, into nursing homes and other care facilities. The narrative that aging is shameful and youthfulness is revered is also reinforced in the way we examine the past. Much of the scholarship in bioarchaeology focuses on individuals who died young or during their peak reproductive years; far fewer researchers examine the remains of individuals who lived into old age. A reframed attention to the experiences of those living into old age may offer a glimpse into larger social frameworks of identity, beliefs, and cultural practices, as well as physical resiliency over the course of a long life.

This chapter offers a biocultural perspective on the experiences of aging women in the Victorian era. We consider the female body and its physiology as well as the social and cultural ways in which women were seen during in their post-reproductive years. From menopause to mourning and death, we move through this experience by placing the limited, but nonetheless useful, bioarchaeological studies alongside scholarship that includes primary sources and the voices of Victorian women themselves. It is particularly hard to understand the lived experience of the aging female body, as we often do not study or analyze this time of life. Yet, if a Victorian woman survived to adulthood and through her childbearing years, she was likely to live into old age, which at the time could be anywhere past the age of 60. Thus, the idea that prior to the twentieth century and the advent of "modern" medicine and changes in living standards, people were likely to die young, misrepresents the reality of lived experience.

In this chapter, we argue that Victorian women, who were likelier to outlive their male counterparts, experienced a range of both physiological and social changes as they aged. These changes included the effects of menopause, which was a subject of ongoing research in the era and was considered a turning point for women's physical and mental health and well-being. For Victorian women experiencing menopause, the change in their reproductive status affected perceptions of their role, both within the family and in the broader societal context. The figure of the Victorian widow, although not representative of the diversity of older women's life experiences, became a symbol of the ritualized culture around mourning and death that characterized the era. There is much to be learned from turning our focus to the bodies and lives of older women in the Victorian period. This neglected field of scholarship offers rich possibilities for further research.

## *Aging: Demographics of Old Age in Victorian England*

Before examining the lived experience of older Victorian women, it is important to understand the demographics of aging, and how aging has been considered within scholarship in anthropology and social history. Methods used to assess demographics, and more specifically mortality rates as well as life expectancy, normally rely on statistics. For mortality demographics today, the Centers for Disease Control (CDC) rely on data collected from the National Vital Statistics System, which is generated by each state recording all deaths on an annual basis. This practice of data collection underpins the operation of modern public health systems. But in the nineteenth century, these systems were in their infancy. The recording of vital statistics was decentralized and not standardized. Church records were often where births and deaths were recorded, but as the century progressed, these data were shifting to hospitals and becoming part of the public record, particularly in urban settings. Scholars therefore need to look to a range of source material for information on patterns of aging, morbidity, and mortality.

Most of the information on morbidity and mortality patterns in Victorian England derives from the national vital registration system, which began in 1837 and was largely used in cities (McNay et al. 2005). This method of data collection presents some clear problems, as life and death outside of the city are often not part of the discussion, and individuals who were counted tend to be those who passed through the public health system; our information is therefore incomplete. What we do know is that there was an overall decline in mortality rates in England as the nineteenth century progressed (Woods and Hinde 1987). This decline is typically attributed to changes in living conditions, diet, housing, sanitary and public health laws, and medical progress in understanding disease transmission and other wellness factors (Woods and Hinde 1987; Hardy 1988). While each of these factors was important in the reduction of morbidity and mortality, we need to remember that the era's high rates of morbidity and mortality were caused by decades, if not centuries, of poor living conditions. Further, as the industrial revolution took hold, disparities between rich and poor increased, as did the health issues related to living in urban environments.

Assessing demographic trends such as *life expectancy* (the expected age of death in a given population) can be complicated by the lack of a centralized data repository. Therefore our understandings of demographic patterns are reliant on archaeological assessments, which only have access to a sample of the dead for a particular time. In addition, when we discuss life expectancy, we need to remind ourselves that we are focusing on "the *average age* to which a member of a cohort can live; the members of a cohort being those born into a specified population at a given time" (Pavelka and Fedigan 1991, 15). Such statistical analysis can be affected by other factors; for example, if there is high infant mortality within a particular community, life expectancy will diminish dramatically. We need to consider the complexity of this type of measurement, as it is highly influenced by environmental variables.

By contrast to life expectancy, when we examine *life span* we refer to the actual age at death for members of a particular cohort. So even in a historical period in which life expectancy might be low, life spans could actually be high, if individuals were able to make it through critical life events: birth, infancy, and childhood, and in the case of female life spans, pregnancy and childbirth. Today, the average life expectancy of women in the industrialized world is currently set at 82 years for females and 76 years for males, whereas the maximum life span is estimated to be somewhere between 100 and 115 years (Duffin 2019). For the Victorian woman, life expectancy was low: in 1841 it has been assessed at around 42.2 (40.2 for males) and by the end of the Victorian period (1900) this had improved to 52.4 for females (48.5 for males) (McNay et al. 2005). Mortality data reveal an excess of death for females as compared to males: even though women were living longer on average, they died at higher rates than men (McNay et al. 2005). These disparities are often attributed to the assumed hazards of childbirth, as well as the idea that female bodies are less hardy than their male counterparts. But the contributing factors are far more complex and are fraught with biocultural intersections that are hard to untangle. As we have discussed, one example is the impact of chronic health issues that were socially constructed and exacerbated by changes in the environment, such as the epidemic of rickets together with corset use. But is also clear that over the course of an individual's life, there were many factors that could cause illness and death, ranging from the medical (chronic health conditions and disease) to the social and cultural (industrial accidents and cultural practices now known to be damaging to the health, such as smoking and excessive alcohol use).

For Victorian women who made it past the critical periods that could cause untimely death (birth, childhood, and reproduction), the odds were good that they would live into old age. Leaving behind their reproductive roles and shifting into midlife and aging meant a shift in physiology (menopause) and a change in social status depending on whether one was unmarried (spinsterhood) or married (widowhood). Even in this era, women tended to outlive men, and therefore were likelier to experience the health and social circumstances incumbent on old age.

## Victorian Women at Midlife

### *A Biocultural Perspective on Menopause*

Menopause, often termed the "change of life," is most often understood as the post-reproductive years. Today, clinically, we recognize menopause as officially beginning when the menstrual cycle has stopped for one year, referring to the time prior to this as the pre-menopause and perimenopause phases, in which the body is adjusting to hormonal changes and a decline in fertility (Pavelka and Fedigan 1991). This period is called the climacteric, a term often used interchangeably with pre- and perimenopause (Pavelka and Fedigan 1991; Davis et al. 2005). Human reproductive senescence, which is the decline in the reproductive system, is only one aspect of the changes that occur, but it tends to be the one we can focus on as it represents a shift in the roles often associated with women's lived experience, from entering the reproductive years to becoming a matriarch. Needless to say, not all Victorian women experienced motherhood, but menopause was a physiological change that affected almost all aging female bodies.

Physiologically, the premenopausal or perimenopausal period is the time that the body's hormonal processes, which since adolescence had been geared towards ovulation (egg release from the ovaries), are preparing to shut down. The human reproductive cycle, beginning at the start of menstruation, usually ends around age 50, with a median age between 40 and 50 years (Gosden 1985; Pavelka and Fedigan 1991). As discussed earlier in this text, female reproduction presents a costly strain on the physical body, and the caloric intake needed for pregnancy and birth as well as the physical strain directly on the body is best undertaken during the prime reproductive years, which are roughly 16–30. When the physical body begins to slow its fertility around age 35–40, the climacteric phase begins. Prior to modern biomedical understanding of these physiological processes, the symptoms of menopause were recognized as part of the aging process for Victorian female bodies.

The physical symptoms of menopause have been recognized across time. Most researchers cite Aristotle's (384–322 BCE) acknowledgement of the onset of menopause, in which he notes that menstruation ends for women at age 40. However, the term "menopause" was not used until the nineteenth century, when it was officially recognized as a medical syndrome in an 1816 French journal article by C. P. L. de Gardanne, "De la Ménopause" (published as a book in 1821). Dating back centuries, however, there were numerous remedies catalogued and used by women to help manage the symptoms of menopause resulting from hormonal changes. These symptoms can include: irregular periods, hot flashes, night sweats, irritability, poor sleep, vaginal dryness, and a sense of sadness or depression. While the onset, duration, and actual symptoms vary from one individual to another and across cultures, Victorian social ideals suggest that this transition was again a charged time for women. In the Victorian period, as Smith-Rosenberg notes, "menopause was seen as a physiological crisis, its course shaped by a woman's preceding sexual experiences, its resolution determining her future health" (1973, 65). Further, the symptoms of menopause were also misunderstood, as it was thought that cessation of menstruation resulted in the retention of the monthly blood within the body, which was believed to cause health issues and mental disorders (Smith-Rosenberg 1973; Showalter 1985; Shuttleworth 1990; Davis et al. 2005).

The aging process for both men and women comes with a number of skeletal markers, most commonly a reduction in bone density (osteoporosis), arthritic changes in the joints, and a loss or wearing away of dentition. Until recently the physiological changes that occur with menopause, much like those associated with menstruation, seemed to have no clear skeletal markers. But a 2016 study by Huseynov and colleagues, using computed 3D tomography (CT) scans of 275 known individuals (151 males and 124 females) ranging in age from developing infants to 95 years old, discovered that there are structural changes of the pelvis over the life span that occur in direct response to reproductive hormones. As noted in Chapter 3, research shows that the pelvis is at its peak obstetrical size between 25 to 30 years of age. While, Huseynov and colleagues' 3D animations of pelvis revealed that "[a]round the age of 40–45, the female pelvis resumes a mode of shape change which is similar to that of males" (2016, 5229). Interestingly, much of the research done on the bony structures of the pelvis has been focused on sexual dimorphism, in particular on the age-related changes of puberty and parturition; this is the first study to examine changes in the post-reproductive period, and it suggests new directions for research into skeletal evidence of aging and changes in sexual dimorphism.

Medical and biological arguments related to menopause in the Victorian era resulted in a focus on the larger systemic issues around female wellness and illness (Stolberg 1999). The French physician Charles F. Ponsan de Menville's 1839 book *Histoire médicale et philosophique de la femme considerée dans toutes les époques principales de sa vie* (*Medical and Philosophical History of Woman Considered in All the Principle Stages of Her Life*) perpetuated the assumption that menopause resulted from the death of the womb. By the end of the Victorian era, developing scientific perspectives on menopause saw it as a syndrome that needed attention, and it became part of the suite of mental health issues that were thought to afflict women. In an 1899 article entitled "Epochal Insanities," Dr. T. S. Clouston described a condition he termed "Climacteric Insanity," arguing that "when the power to reproduce ceases, the whole vital energy is lessened, and begins to shew [sic] signs of decay."[1] This state of physiological decay, linked to the cessation of menstruation, was seen as a root cause for an increase in mental health issues, which were thought to include a heightened sense of melancholy or depression, restlessness, delusions, and even suicidal tendencies. Clouston's (1899) suggested treatments reflect some methods still in use today to address the hormonal changes associated with menopause, but also included blood-letting to release the retained blood and some substances now known to be toxic: his range of recommendations included "fresh air [...] careful dieting, frequent meals of stimulating as well as nourishing food, wines and malt liquors used dietetically, the natural mineral waters, quinine, iron, strychnine, the hypophosphites, arsenic, and other tonics" (935).[2] In the Victorian period, then, menopause was seen as a condition to be ameliorated by medical intervention, rather than a natural bodily process. Modern research has shown that menopause is not linked to mental illness, and some progress has been made in the way doctors now approach the physical symptoms of menopause; however, many cultural assumptions remain in place regarding the "change of life" and its effects on women's lives.

### *Cultural Perceptions*

As Kay Heath notes in her study of aging in the nineteenth century, and as we discuss in Chapter 4, Victorian women were defined by their ability to reproduce—or in the words of Pat Jalland and John Hooper, through their roles as "potential mothers, actual mothers, or retired mothers" (Heath 2009, 15, citing Jalland and Hooper 1986, 5). Women who remained unmarried at age 30 were expected to resign themselves to spinsterhood and were often caricatured in fiction and in the popular press as desexualized, desiccated, or to use the dominant metaphor of the era, flowers whose bloom had withered (Matus 1995). Since women were defined through their reproductive capacity, "from their mid-forties, when they were considered menopausal, women were depicted as increasingly less valuable" (Heath 2009, 15).

The English physician Edward John Tilt published the first British treatise on menopause, *The Change of Life in Woman, in Health and Disease*, in 1857. This text addresses female physiology at the "decline of life" and the diseases that Tilt thought could be exacerbated or remediated by the cessation of menstruation. Tilt argued that menopause renders both body and mind more "masculine" (1857, 25), a claim based on Victorian assumptions about marked gender differences in both physical and mental characteristics as well as behavior. A similar claim was promulgated in the 1870s by John Braxton Hicks, who first identified the pre-labor uterine contractions with which his name is now associated: he argued that menopausal women "revert to the neutral man-woman state," becoming effectively sexless once their menses have ceased (Braxton Hicks 1877, 475). As they aged, Victorian women therefore contended with a complex set of gendered assumptions and discourses that linked their cultural and social status to a biologically deterministic view of gender as defined through sex, and particularly through reproduction.

Victorian novels, particularly the works of Charles Dickens, are rife with satirical representations of women at midlife and beyond. Older women in these fictions are depicted as subjects for comic ridicule at best (the widowed Mrs. Sparsit in *Hard Times*), and objects of pitiable horror at worst (the elderly spinster Miss Havisham in *Great Expectations*). However, writers such as Elizabeth Gaskell, in her 1853 novel *Cranford*, countered the stereotype of the withered, nagging, or ineffectual older woman in characterizing elderly spinsters and widows as gentle, loving, and productive members of society. The Victorian widow is an especially complex figure who symbolizes both the centrality of domesticity and family to the lives of married women, and the legal, economic, and social ramifications of widowhood for women's lives.

## The Victorian Widow

Statistically, more women were widowed than men in the nineteenth century, and men were more likely to remarry. As Pat Jalland observes in *Death in the Victorian Family*, "after 1850 the number of widows over 35 in England and Wales was more than double that of widowers" (1996, 230). The resulting demographic realities had reverberating effects on the daily lives and cultural perceptions of widows in the Victorian period. Women who did not remarry after a spouse's death had lost the culturally valued role of wife and were set apart from society, marked in visible ways. However, once her husband died, a woman was no longer considered *feme covert*, and benefited from greater legal freedoms than unmarried women or married women with husbands still living (Smith 1854; Shanley 1989).

By comparison to widowers, who were expected to return to work soon after a spouse's death and who were culturally permitted to remarry at an earlier date, Victorian widows struggled with "the total disintegration of their lives" (Jalland 1996, 235) that could result from financial instability contingent on the absence of the primary wage-earner, loss of status and occupation, and sometimes a literal sense of displacement if they had to change residences or sell their belongings to make ends meet. Middle-class widows left without sources of financial support had few options other than teaching, and working-class widows had to balance the demands of child-rearing and the management of the home with the necessity of returning to work or seeking employment. Surveys conducted by Charles Booth and Benjamin Seebohm Rowntree in working-class urban districts in London and York found that the lowest income category was primarily made up of families who had lost the income of the primary (male) breadwinner; widows were also among the likeliest recipients of poor relief (Strange 2005). The Old Age Pensions Act was not passed until 1908; before that time, pensions were not guaranteed, and even wealthy women were reliant on family members for settlements and annuities.

One especially interesting example is the role played by Queen Victoria in constructing cultural perceptions of widowhood during this period (Figure 5.1). Queen Victoria's widowhood cast a shadow over the nation in 1861, when Prince Albert died of typhoid fever at age 42. Queen Victoria sought seclusion for a longer period of time than was usual, withdrawing as much as possible from her official duties. In her letters, she expressed the intensity of her grief: "To lose one's partner in life is [...] like losing *half* of one's *body* and *soul* [...] But to the Queen—to a poor helpless woman—it is not that only—it is the stay, support and comfort which is lost! To the Queen it is like *death* in life!" (Queen Victoria to Earl Canning, 10 January 1862, *Letters of Queen Victoria*, Vol. III, 608). The queen famously wore mourning dress for the remaining 40 years of her life, and her black gowns and widow's cap have become enduring images of Victorian widowhood, despite the fact that such lengthy and chronic expressions of grief were atypical for the era.

As we elaborate at greater length below, Victorian widows were expected to show their devotion to their dead husbands by following some of the strictest mourning requirements. They sought consolation in religious observance, surviving family, and keeping the memory of the loved

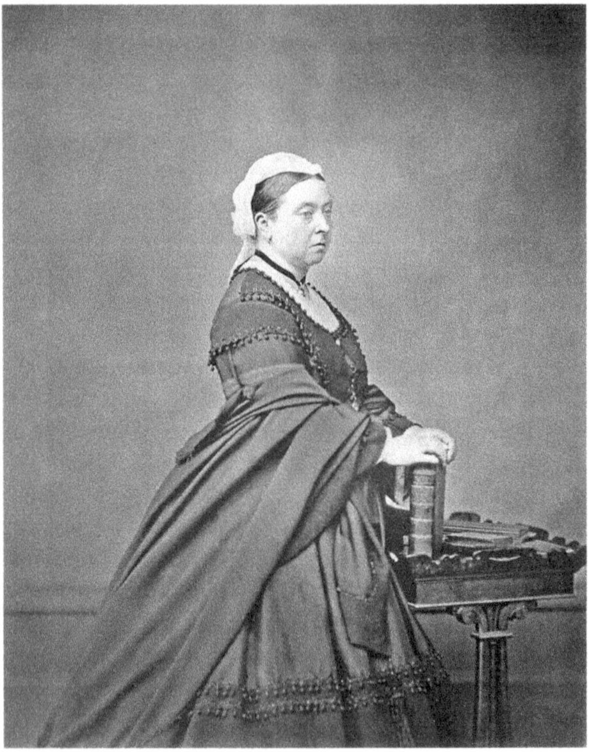

*Figure 5.1* Queen Victoria. Credit: Wellcome Collection. https://wellcomecollection.org/works/ty2m6shb

one alive. Many of these modes of observance were shared by Victorians regardless of gender or class; but others were distinguished by the age, gender, class, and social position of the individuals and family members of the dead. In the next section, we explore some of the many rituals and practices associated with death, dying, and memorialization in the nineteenth century.

### *Death and Dying in the Nineteenth Century*

As Julie-Marie Strange notes in her study of death, grief, and poverty in the late nineteenth and early twentieth centuries, "material circumstances were integral to the manner in which families dealt with the dead" (2005, 11). For the observant, death was viewed through a religious lens: the Evangelical revival had a tremendous influence over the way death was conceived in the nineteenth century, in turn shaping the Protestant ideal of the "good death" (Jalland 1996, 26). In contrast to sudden deaths, which did not allow the dying to ready themselves for the experience of death, the "good death" enabled a degree of psychological and practical preparation. Under this model, even if dying itself was a trial, the ideal was to submit to God's will, with the promise of a reunion with loved ones after death. The opposite experiences were dreaded—not just the "bad death" that might result from physical suffering, but also sudden deaths and suicides for which the family had little time to prepare (Jalland 1996; Strange 2005). In an increasingly secular population, agnostics and atheists coped with death in different ways, viewing it as inevitable, but also experiencing feelings of bitterness and in some cases confronting existential questions about the meaning (or meaninglessness of) human existence.

Women were centrally involved in death, particularly in their culturally accepted role as nurses and caretakers. In literary and artistic representations, Victorian wives, mothers, and daughters were often depicted at the bedsides of beloved family members, demonstrating both the patient endurance and the heightened emotions associated with the loss of a loved one. Death was also a task that fell to female domestic servants and, after the 1870s, trained sick nurses (Jalland 1996). When a family member died (usually at home), the blinds were drawn or curtains closed, mirrors were covered, and the body was laid out by nurses and/or female servants (Jalland 1996; Strange 2005; Frisby 2015). Women played a vital role in caring for the corpse and assuring respect for the dead, even as there was increasing cultural investment in professionalizing the treatment of the dead by undertakers (Strange 2005; Henry 2016).

With respect to the rituals associated with death such as funeral rites and burial services, there were divisions in the etiquette and grandeur of ceremonies according to class. However, as the century progressed, Victorians expressed a growing preference for "simple and dignified ceremonies" (Jalland 1996, 200) rather than the opulence and extravagance associated with the most elaborate state funerals such as that of the Duke of Wellington in 1852 (Pearsall 1999). Especially among the poor and working classes, most funeral rites "cost little and were often improvised" (Strange 2005, 23), although families were loath to sacrifice the idea of a proper service that would treat the dead with dignity and respect.

In the 1870s, undertaking firms offered a range of services ranging from modest to extravagant funerals. For the upper and middle classes, the funeral could be an elaborate formal procession, with a coach drawn by horses with black plumes, and a coffin draped in black, carried by male servants or an undertaker's employees. Male family members attended the funeral service at the church and the burial service at the graveyard or cemetery. Given the predominance of the Church of England, the Anglican burial service was widely used for the latter; the Burial Act of 1880 made it possible for Catholics and Nonconformists to have a service led by a minister of their choice, although the dead would be located in Anglican burial grounds (Wiggins 1996; Strange 2005). Women typically remained at home, whether from perceptions that they could not control their expressions of grief, or were more emotionally vulnerable; in working-class families, women might remain at home for similar reasons of perceived propriety, but also to prepare the funeral tea (Strange 2005; Frisby 2015). Alternatively, working-class families might have "walking funerals" in which friends of the family served as pallbearers; often they contributed funds toward organizations that would pay for the member's burial expenses (Mitchell 1996). It was of paramount importance to avoid the stigma of a pauper burial (and its association with the workhouse and with fees being paid by the parish rather than the family) by observing the rites associated with a proper commemoration of the dead: "The vast majority of bereaved families participated in death rites which were not only expected performances of mourning, but were also imbued with shared understandings of decency, dignity, custom, and respectability" (Strange 2005, 26). Late nineteenth-century debates over cremation and the public mortuary movement underscored the concern with proper recognition and memorialization of the dead (Jalland 1996; Murdoch 2015).

The transition between the death of a loved one and the grieving process was understandably difficult, and the etiquette of mourning (described in detail in the next section) allowed community members to recognize the death and its impact (Frisby 2015). In her study of elite Victorian families, Patricia Jalland describes the "funeral week" as "a hiatus between nursing the dying and the prolonged period of individual grieving" (Jalland 1996, 210). Families memorialized their dead through paintings, photographs, drawings, busts, and silhouettes; many of these likenesses were made during the dead person's life, but others were made after death, as a way to remember the physical appearance of the dead person. The investment in a physical memento of the dead extended to the phenomenon of death-masks, which were made immediately after death from plaster casts of the face, head and shoulders, and hands (Jalland 1996). Family members and friends of the deceased participated in the communal rituals of mourning and recognition through floral tributes, visits to the gravesite, and letters of condolence and remembrance. When individuals had time to plan for their own deaths, they not only laid out their wishes in writing through wills and commemorative bequests, but also relied on informal methods of communication about their intentions for valued objects (sentimental or otherwise). Prior to the Married Women's Property Acts of 1870 and 1882, women were unable to make wills of their own, since they had no independent legal existence; therefore such informal modes of communication were essential in order to convey their intentions to family members. One of the most common ways of commemorating the dead was to retain a lock of their hair as a keepsake; and in some cases, such commemorative keepsakes would be passed on to subsequent generations. Victorian hair jewelry remains a powerfully evocative and tangible symbol of the ways in which the dead were materially remembered by the living (Nehama 2012; Swindle 2017).

### *The Etiquette of Mourning: Codes and Practices*

Regardless of class, following the death of a relative or close friend, Victorians participated in a culturally prescribed set of mourning practices, of which there were many specific features and guidelines. In wealthier families, black-edged stationery announced the death, and major events would be curtailed or cancelled altogether until a suitable period of time had passed. Widows were not expected to accept formal invitations or appear in public for the first year of their two-year period of formal mourning. For other family members, the mourning period was lessened: a year for parent or child, six months for a sibling. The attire of family members signaled that the family was in mourning, and allowed others to understand any reticence to participate in social functions. The upper classes would keep an entirely separate wardrobe for mourning; middle- and working-class people adapted existing garments, dying them black or otherwise economizing for the period of observance (Strange 2005).

Gendered distinctions in clothing meant that men modified their clothing less than women; nonetheless they wore specific mourning garments including black armbands, gloves, hatbands, and/or cravats. Women, particularly wives, mothers, and daughters, wore dresses made from bombazine, crêpe (sometimes spelled crape), or other dull fabrics. Widows were expected to wear full mourning or "weeds" for two years, with dresses made from "non-reflective black paramatta [a twill fabric made from silk or cotton and wool] and crape for the first year of deepest mourning, followed by nine months of dullish black silk, heavily trimmed with crape, and then three months when crape was discarded" (Jalland 1996, 300). Widows' caps, and veils for outdoors, were worn for the first year, though could be worn much longer. Depending on the degree of formality observed, after a period of six months or a year, female family members could transition to half-mourning in shades of grey or lavender. A 2014–2015 exhibition at New York's Metropolitan Museum of Art presented a number of examples of full and half-mourning, including gowns worn by Queen Victoria and Queen Alexandra ("Death Becomes Her," Metropolitan Museum of Art, New York).

After the first stages of deep mourning, women of the upper and middle classes would wear jewelry made from jet, a gemstone derived from fossilized wood; the coastal region of Whitby in North Yorkshire was a popular source for jet jewelry in the nineteenth century. Victorians also popularized the tradition of wearing bracelets, brooches, and pendants made from the woven hair of the deceased, encased behind glass (Nehama 2012) (Figure 5.2).

Although perceptions of the rigid codes and practices associated with mourning in the nineteenth century have been somewhat exaggerated, it is certainly the case that Victorians considered it essential to observe the rituals of mourning, and these extended to the deaths of prominent figures throughout the century. Sally Mitchell notes that "When Queen Victoria died, almost everyone in England wore black for three months" (Mitchell 1996, 163). The Victorian commitment to propriety, tradition,

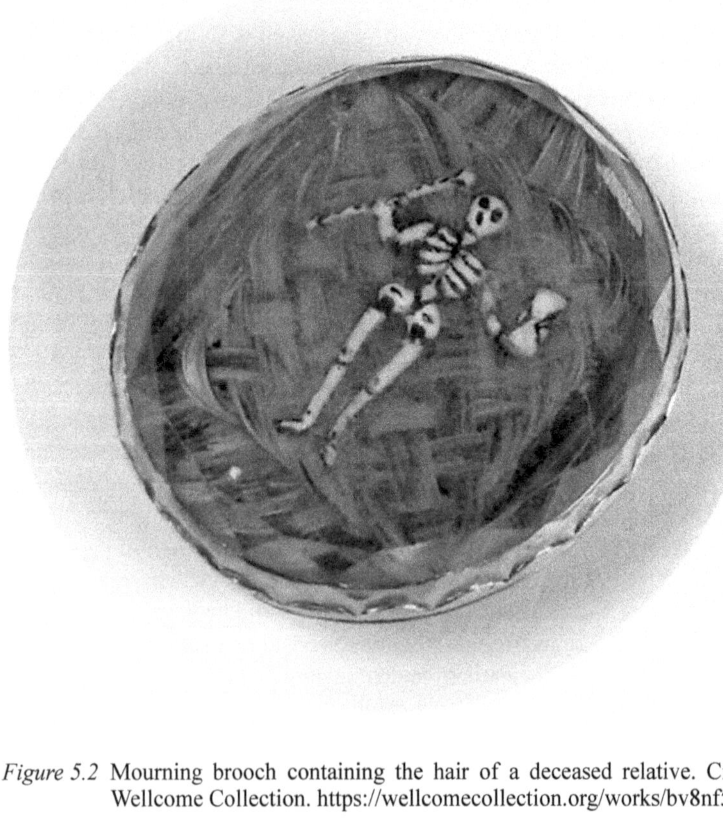

*Figure 5.2* Mourning brooch containing the hair of a deceased relative. Credit: Wellcome Collection. https://wellcomecollection.org/works/bv8nf5qy

and observance meant that mourning practices were a cultural form that united people in a recognition of the lives of those who had died, and the symbolic endurance of Victorian mourning rituals speaks to the cultural significance of the closing years of an individual's life. Recent scholarship has deepened our understanding of aging and senescence from both cultural and bioarchaeological perspectives, and suggest new paths for further research into this less studied but fascinating time in the lives of Victorian women.

## To Sum Up

- Late in life, women's bodies and lives begin to accommodate different realities of lived experience, not only the dominant reproductive model.
- Victorian scientists began to identify the physical effects of menopause and aging on the older woman's body; however, their perceptions continued to be structured by nineteenth-century ideologies of sex and gender difference.
- Women were likelier to outlive men in the Victorian period, leading to a range of cultural representations of aging spinsters and widows, who played an important societal role in a ritualized culture of mourning.

## Notes

1 This article includes a section delineating states of insanity during each reproductive period for females including: *The Insanity of Pregnancy and Adolescents*, *The Insanity of Pregnancy*, and *Lactational Insanity* (Clouston 1899).

2 *Hypophosphites* (phosphinates) were used in patent medicines and tonics throughout the nineteenth century; for an example, see Fellows 1881. Arsenic is known to be poisonous in large doses but was thought to be medically beneficial in certain circumstances, as on this list of potential treatments; for more on the medical use of arsenic in the nineteenth century, see Whorton 2010.

## References

### *Primary Sources*

Braxton-Hicks, J. 1877. "The Croonian Lectures on the Difference Between the Sexes in Regard to the Aspect and Treatment of Disease." *British Medical Journal* 1 (851): 475–476.

Clouston, T. S. 1899. "Epochal Insanities." *A System of Medicine* 8: 926–941.

De Gardanne, Charles Pierre Louis. 1821. *De la ménopause: ou, de l'age critique des femmes*. 2nd ed. Paris: Méquignon-Marvis.

De Menville, Charles F. Ponsan. 1845. *Histoire médicale et philosophique de la femme considerée dans toutes les époques principales de sa vie*. Paris: Chez L'Auteur, Rue Saint-Honore.

Dickens, Charles. 1861. *Great Expectations*. Edited with an introduction by Graham Law and Adrian J. Pinnington. Peterborough, ON: Broadview Press, 1998.

Dickens, Charles. 1854. *Hard Times*. Edited with an introduction by Kate Flint. London/New York: Penguin, 2007.

Fellows, James I. 1881. *A Few Remarks upon Fellows' Hypophosphites of Quinine, Strychnine, Iron, Lime, Potassa, and Manganese*. London: Jas. I. Fellows.

Gaskell, Elizabeth. 1853. *Cranford*. Edited with an introduction by Patricia Ingham. London/New York: Penguin Classics, 2005.

Smith, Barbara Leigh [later Bodichon]. 1854. 2nd ed. revised with additions, 1856. *A Brief Summary, in Plain Language, of the Most Important Laws Concerning Women; Together with a Few Observations Thereon*. London: John Chapman.

### *Secondary Sources*

Davis, Susan Ruth, I. Dinatale, L. Rivera-Woll, and Sonia Davison. 2005. "Postmenopausal Hormone Therapy: From Monkey Glands to Transdermal Patches." *Journal of Endocrinology* 185 (2): 207–222.

Frisby, Helen. 2015. "Drawing the Pillow, Laying Out and Port Wine: The Moral Economy of Death, Dying and Bereavement in England, c.1840–1930." *Mortality* 20 (2): 103–127.

Gosden, R. G. 1985. *Biology of Menopause. The Cause and Consequence of Ovarian Ageing*. London: Academic Press.

Hardy, Anne. 1988. "Diagnosis, Death, and Diet: The Case of London, 1750–1909." *The Journal of Interdisciplinary History* 18 (3): 387–401.

Heath, Kay. 2009. *Aging by the Book: The Emergence of Midlife in Victorian Britain*. Albany, NY: State University of New York Press.

Henry, Wanda S. 2016. "Women Searchers of the Dead in Eighteenth- and Nineteenth-Century London." *Social History of Medicine* 29 (3): 445–466.

Huseynov, Alik, Christoph P. E. Zollikofer, Walter Coudyzer, Dominic Gascho, Christian Kellenberger, Ricarda Hinzpeter, and Marcia S. Ponce de León. 2016. "Developmental Evidence for Obstetric Adaptation of the Human Female Pelvis." *Proceedings of the National Academy of Sciences* 113 (19): 5227–5232.

Jalland, Pat. 1996. *Death in the Victorian Family*. Oxford: Oxford University Press.

Jalland, Pat, and John Hooper. 1986. *Women from Birth to Death: The Female Life Cycle in Britain, 1830–1914*. Atlantic Highlands, NJ: Humanities Press International.

Matus, Jill. 1995. *Unstable Bodies: Victorian Representations of Sexuality and Maternity*. Manchester/New York: Manchester University Press.

McNay, Kirsty, Jane Humphries, and Stephan Klasen. 2005. "Excess Female Mortality in Nineteenth-Century England and Wales: A Regional Analysis." *Social Science History* 29 (4): 649–681.

Mitchell, Sally. 1996. *Daily Life in Victorian England.* Westport, CT: Greenwood Press.

Murdoch, Lydia. 2015. "'The Dead and the Living': Child Death, the Public Mortuary Movement, and the Spaces of Grief and Selfhood in Victorian London." *Journal of the History of Childhood & Youth* 8 (3): 378–402.

Nehama, Sarah. 2012. *In Death Lamented: The Tradition of Anglo-American Mourning Jewelry*. Boston, MA: Massachusetts Historical Society.

Pavelka, Mary S. M., and Linda Marie Fedigan. 1991. "Menopause: A Comparative Life History Perspective." *American Journal of Physical Anthropology* 34 (S13): 13–38.

Pearsall, Cornelia D. J. 1999. "Burying the Duke: Victorian Mourning and the Funeral of the Duke of Wellington." *Victorian Literature and Culture* 27 (2): 365–393.

Shanley, Mary Lyndon. 1989. *Feminism, Marriage and the Law in Victorian England, 1850–1895*. Princeton, NJ: Princeton University Press.

Showalter, Elaine. 1985. *The Female Malady: Women, Madness, and English Culture, 1830–1980*. New York: Penguin.

Shuttleworth, Sally. 1990. "Female Circulation: Medical Discourse and Popular Advertising in the Mid-Victorian Era." In *Body/Politics: Women and the Discourses of Science*, edited by Mary Jacobus, Evelyn Fox Keller, and Sally Shuttleworth, 47–68. New York: Routledge.

Smith-Rosenberg, Carroll. 1973. "Puberty to Menopause: The Cycle of Femininity in Nineteenth-Century America." *Feminist Studies* 1 (3/4): 58–72.

Stolberg, Michael. 1999. "A Woman's Hell? Medical Perceptions of Menopause in Preindustrial Europe." *Bulletin of the History of Medicine* 73 (3): 404–428.

Strange, Julie-Marie. 2005. *Death, Grief and Poverty in Britain, 1870–1914*. Cambridge: Cambridge University Press.

Swindle, Lanah. 2017. "'Keep this as a Small Token of Love': A Brief History of British and American Hair Jewelry." Unpublished independent study project supervised by Professor Sura Levine. Amherst, MA: Hampshire College.

Whorton, James C. 2010. *The Arsenic Century: How Victorian Britain Was Poisoned at Home, Work, and Play*. Oxford: Oxford University Press.

Wiggins, Deborah. 1996. "The Burial Act of 1880, the Liberation Society and George Osborne Morgan." *Parliamentary History* 15 (2): 173–189.

Woods, Robert, and P. R. Andrew Hinde. 1987. "Mortality in Victorian England: Models and Patterns." *Journal of Interdisciplinary History* 18 (1): 27–54.

### *Online Resources*

Metropolitan Museum of Art. "Death Becomes Her." Exhibition at the Metropolitan Museum of Art, New York, New York. 2014–2015. https://www.metmuseum.org/exhibitions/listings/2014/death-becomes-her/gallery-views. Accessed 31 July 2019.

Duffin, Erin. 2019. "Average Life Expectancy in Industrial and Developing Countries for Those Born in 2018, by Gender (in Years)." Population Reference Bureau Release date, August 2018. https://www.statista.com/statistics/274507/life-expectancy-in-industrial-and-developing-countries/. Accessed 11 September 2019.

# 6 Victorian Bodies, Modern Issues

## Conclusions: Science and Culture Revisited

In undertaking this investigation of women's bodies and lives in the Victorian era, we have benefited from an interdisciplinary approach that brings together science and culture in new ways. Recent scholarship in a variety of fields has already begun to explore the productive intersections arising from combining, for example, the study of literature and the history of science; new areas of inquiry such as ecological criticism have facilitated a deeper understanding of Victorian environmental change (MacDuffie 2014; Hall 2017; Williams 2017). In working with a dual focus on science and culture, we have striven to bring a new set of questions to bear on each field, looking at scientific texts from the perspective of their cultural production, and examining culture with a scientific lens. Our project underscores that culture and biology are not separate spheres; they are intersectional and multidimensional.

A biocultural approach affords a rich interpretation of the past, because it allows scholars to cross disciplinary boundaries in order to consider the lived experience of Victorian women from multiple perspectives (social, biological, political—to name only a few). We were trained and teach in distinct disciplines—areas traditionally separated into "the sciences" and "the humanities"—but through our collaborative research, writing, and teaching, we have learned a great deal about how these areas of inquiry can be placed in conversation. Analytical methods involving everything from archival research in women's history to the analysis of skeletal remains, and ranging from the history of medicine and science to the study of fashion, empire and colonization, and the novel—each of these approaches to scholarship has benefited from a dual perspective on the Victorian period integrating the questions and modes of inquiry of our disciplines. This model has also enabled us to develop a deeper understanding of what is present and absent in the historical record, and has informed our suggestions for further research and questions to consider at the end of each chapter.

Although we each come at the practice of historical study with different perspectives, and believe that this project offers a unique opportunity for synthesis, we recognize that this is not the only approach to this material; it is a window into the "how" rather than a limitation on the "what" of our analysis. We hope that readers of this text—from undergraduate students embarking on the study of the Victorian era or biocultural studies for the first time, to more experienced scholars and students—will be inspired to add to this study, to analyze additional evidence where it may be found, and to expand and enrich our understanding of the period.

## Contemporary Relevance

While we have thought a great deal about the past and interpretations that can be made from a variety of entry points about women's lives in the Victorian era, we also see this work as important in understanding systems of oppression and the workings of privilege and power today. Of necessity, given the historical evidence, our study has concentrated primarily on white European women, and how their bodies have been used as sites in which behavior and biology were policed by patriarchal ideology. This is the way historical analyses and bioarchaeological studies most often position themselves. The research develops from a dominant, white, and male perspective, which shapes the primary source material that in turn leads to scientific and historical documentation produced during the period and afterward. In these narratives there is little mention of non-white people, or when they are mentioned it is because researchers chose to study those on the margins; but marginalization is the product of imperialism and cultural dominance. As noted in Chapter 1, for example, there is a paucity of scholarship on women of color in the Victorian period, except in the context of the ways in which they were rendered erotic or exotic, as bodies to be dissected by medicine and put on display for public view. In fact it is the Victorian era that solidifies racial and gendered differences as real, rigid, and unchanging.

### *Science and the Normal White Female Body*

The framing of the "normal white female body" finds its roots in developing evolutionary thought, scientific theories of racial and gender difference, and Victorian codes of proper femininity. As we note in Chapter 2, there was a clear focus on human difference within Victorian science and medicine, originally intertwined with supporting the concept of the "great chain of being" (Gilman 1985, 212) and the search to solidify polygenetic origins, and used to make medical assessments and undertake skeletal analyses. The Victorian era plays a pivotal role in shaping how scientific texts, and subsequently modern anthropological studies, frame the concept of the "normal body," and this framing continues to be used without interrogation. This is the normative model by which all bodies are measured today, in both literal and figurative terms. If we do not recognize and acknowledge the ways in which nineteenth-century science has shaped our understanding of the human experience, we risk reproducing the same flaws and failing to fully understand the complexity of being human.

Imperial and patriarchal ideologies, as we have seen, had a direct impact on the development of race science in the nineteenth century. Underpinning this discourse was the scripted evolutionary narrative of the "civilized" body as the norm by which others were judged. As we have seen, the concept of the "normal white female body" is also predicated on the structural violence fundamental to the cultural performance of beauty for the economically secure and obviously white female, without consideration of the resilient unbound female body in all other contexts. Today, this narrative of normality and deviance persists in subtle ways, devaluing the non-white female body and occluding the operation of power and privilege in constructing systems of oppression that are too often ignored. To remedy the endemic forms of structural violence that masquerade as ideological norms, we need to bring forward the participation of white women (as well as men) in upholding the Victorian standards that now permeate Western medicine. In doing so, we also need to unravel the deeply ingrained ethnocentrism of the nineteenth century and engage in scholarship using a critical white feminist lens that is reflexive and that recognizes the complexity of historical narratives of direct and indirect structural violence, and their influences over how female bodies have been, and continue to be, assessed by science and medicine.

## *Critical White Feminism, Structural Violence, and Victorian Bodies*

A critical white feminist lens, broadly defined, involves "an antiracist transformation of white feminist theory [used] to expand the scope of feminist thought to critically consider whiteness and its privileges by blending aspects of critical white studies and feminist theory to examine power relationships through an intersectional lens" (McFadden 2017, 244). Exploring the Victorian era with the goal of uncovering the ways in which science, social performance, and identity intersect to construct the "normal white" female body, we strive to engage a critical white feminist lens that recognizes the structural violence framework in operation. We acknowledge that examining Victorian ideologies of race and gender can be a form of structural violence, and that we risk reproducing the very norms we seek to reveal. But such scholarship, designed to analyze and expose the workings of racism, class privilege, and other forms of oppression, offers an opportunity to rethink how bodies have become defined as normal or deviant, and how these determinations have been accepted without question. The Victorian construction of the proper, decorous, and restrained female body, whose whiteness is often both assumed and masked, necessitates an evaluation of the historic ways in which female bodies have been privileged or marginalized.

As white feminist scholars ourselves, we need to grapple with the ways in which the structural violence of the Victorian era policed female bodies as it constructed the "normal white female body" as evolved and civilized, above all others (except white men). We need to consider how our own positionality as white women risks reproducing these same ideas, instead of disrupting them. Our challenge is to rethink the history of Victorian race science and the underpinnings of racism that persist today; by looking closely, these practices become visible in their influences and open to interrogation.

Science and biocultural inquiry cannot be absolved of their roles in othering non-white bodies, while simultaneously protecting white bodies. We need to recognize that medicine has a culture of its own—one built on oppression—that must be rethought from an intersectional perspective. To understand what bodies from the past reveal about their time and place, requires not only self-reflection but also a commitment to recognizing our positionality alongside new heuristic contexts. With respect to the study of Victorian culture, this methodology also asks us to engage with interdisciplinary scholarship in critical race theory; recent scholarship by Ronjaunee Chatterjee, Alicia Mireles Christoff, and Amy Wong suggests the potential that lies in this approach.[1] We hope that readers of this text will take up the challenge of analyzing how definitions of sex, gender, and race are culturally contingent and historically scripted, requiring us to consider how our own assumptions may lie at the intersections of the past and present, and helping to shape the future of scholarship in the study of human bodies and lives.

## Note

1 This work was initially presented at the 2019 conferences of the Modern Language Association and the Northeast Victorian Studies Association, and is forthcoming in *Victorian Studies*. We are grateful to Alicia Mireles Christoff for sharing the proposal with us in advance of publication.

## References

Chatterjee, Ronjaunee, Alicia Mireles Christoff, and Amy Wong, eds. 2019. "Critical Theory and the Present of Victorian Studies: A Proposal for a Special Issue of *Victorian Studies*."

Gilman, Sander L. 1985. "Black Bodies, White Bodies: Toward an Iconography of Female Sexuality in Late Nineteenth-Century Art, Medicine, and Literature." *Critical Inquiry* 12 (1): 204–242.

Hall, Dewey W., ed. 2017. *Victorian Ecocriticism: The Politics of Place and Early Environmental Justice*. Lanham, MD: Lexington Books, 2017.

MacDuffie, Allen. 2014. *Victorian Literature, Energy, and the Ecological Imagination.* Cambridge Studies in Nineteenth-Century Literature and Culture: 93. Cambridge: Cambridge University Press.

McFadden, Caroline R. 2017. "Reproductively Privileged: Critical White Feminism and Reproductive Justice Theory." In *Radical Reproductive Justice: Foundations, Theory, Practice, Critique*, edited by Loretta Ross, Erika Derkas, Whitney Peoples, and Pamela Bridgewater, 241–250. New York: The Feminist Press.

Williams, Daniel. 2017. "Victorian Ecocriticism for the Anthropocene." *Victorian Literature & Culture* 45 (3): 667.

# Index

For Product Safety Concerns and Information please contact our EU representative GPSR@taylorandfrancis.com
Taylor & Francis Verlag GmbH, Kaufingerstraße 24, 80331 München, Germany

www.ingramcontent.com/pod-product-compliance
Ingram Content Group UK Ltd.
Pitfield, Milton Keynes, MK11 3LW, UK
UKHW021244190926
475569UK00001BA/4
*9780367026110*